The Public Library
of Nashville
and D........
Co.......

THE
FRAGILE
COALITION

THE
FRAGILE
COALITION

SCIENTISTS, ACTIVISTS, AND AIDS

ROBERT M. WACHTER, M.D.

ASSISTANT PROFESSOR OF MEDICINE
University of California, San Francisco

PROGRAM DIRECTOR
Sixth International Conference on AIDS

St. Martin's Press
NEW YORK

362.1969
W11f

Grateful acknowledgment is made for permission to use the following material:

"On Heaven and Hell." Copyright © Congregation Sha'ar Zahav. Reprinted by permission.

"A Neanderthal Law on AIDS," by Dennis Altman and Andrew Orkin. Copyright © 1989 The New York Times Company. Reprinted by permission.

"A Call to Riot," by Larry Kramer. Copyright © 1990 OutWeek magazine. Reprinted by permission.

Quotations from the speeches and writings of Larry Kramer, collected in Reports from the holocaust: the makings of an AIDS activist. Copyright © 1989 St. Martin's Press. Reprinted by permission.

Unpublished letters by Herbert Daniel, Stephen Joseph, Larry Kramer, Pierre Ludington, Jonathan Mann, Leon McKusick, and Ronald Stall. All are reprinted by permission.

First published in the United States of America in 1991

Printed in the United States of America

ISBN 0-312-05801-2

Library of Congress Cataloging-in-Publication Data

Wachter, Robert M.
    The fragile coalition : scientists, activists, and AIDS / Robert M. Wachter.
        p.   cm.
    ISBN 0-312-05801-2
    1. AIDS (Disease)—Political aspects.   2. International Conference on AIDS.   I. Title.
RC607.A26W33   1991
362.1'969792—dc20   90-27407
                                            CIP

For Bern and Mur, who taught me to listen:
with gratitude, respect, and love

CONTENTS

ACKNOWLEDGMENTS

Although this is a work of nonfiction, it deceives. I fear the reader may be left with the impression that the planning of the Sixth International Conference on AIDS revolved around me alone, with cameo appearances by a half-dozen others. Nothing could be further from the truth. All in all, some seventy-five staff and six hundred volunteers actively participated in the planning of the event. I have never met a more talented and devoted group of people, and do not expect to any time soon. People like Lucy Felicissimo, Dana Van Gorder, Barbara Woodruff, Ben Junge, Erik Jacobson, Judie Weber, Pam Wool, Alice Gruber, David Weisberg, and Dennis Hartzell (to name just a few) were the heart and soul of the effort, and I—and everyone concerned about the AIDS epidemic—owe them a great debt.

Drs. John Ziegler and Paul Volberding, by all rights, should have chosen someone wiser and grayer for my position—though by the end I had become gray enough to almost justify their trust. The support they showed me, and in turn the support and autonomy provided us by University of California, San Francisco Chancellor Julius Krevans, Dean Joseph Martin, Associate Dean Richard Root, the late Dean Richard

Littlejohn, and Chairmen Merle Sande and Floyd Rector, was crucial and appreciated.

I am grateful to Leonard Syme, Professor of Epidemiology at UC Berkeley, for whispering to me in April 1989, "Take good notes, you'll want to write about this when it's over." Drs. Hal Holman and Alan Garber, my mentors at Stanford, backed me all the way while I embarked upon a rather unconventional (to put it mildly) fellowship project; so did the fellowship's sponsors, the Robert Wood Johnson Foundation and the Department of Veterans Affairs. I am also grateful to Drs. Jonathan Mann, June Osborn, Anthony Fauci, Jim Hill, Ken Bridbord, James Allen, Gary Noble, Mervyn Silverman, Jeffrey Harris, and Lars Kallings, all of whom supported me and the conference unstintingly throughout the last two years.

I thank Kermit Hummel, my editor at St. Martin's Press, for his encouragement and his deft touch with a red pencil. Thanks also to Drs. Phil Lee, Bernard Lo, John Luce, Albert Wu, Haya Rubin, and Michael Lesh for their helpful comments on the manuscript.

I learned constantly from the HIV-infected people I met along the way—people like Leon McKusick, Pierre Ludington, Sallie Perryman, Peter Staley, Mike Shriver, Hacib Aoun, and, yes, Larry Kramer. Their dignity, candor, spirit, and intelligence were simply awe-inspiring. Leon was right when, during the opening ceremony of the conference, he observed that much of the anger in this epidemic—shared by activist and scientist alike—is grief, often repressed. That these people may be taken from us prematurely is an inestimable loss and a source of grief to everyone.

Finally, my greatest debt is to my wife Amy, who acted as my personal attorney, editor, public relations director, political advisor, psychotherapist, and best friend during what was a trying time for both of us. Our coalition provides me my greatest source of strength and pride.

PREFACE

This book is about politics. If only it were not so. How different our approach to the catastrophe of AIDS might have been if politicians always led instead of followed, activists always reasoned instead of rioted, scientists always strived for truth instead of prestige, drug companies always pursued cures instead of profits, and journalists always educated instead of titillated.

But, alas, human beings tend to act like human beings, institutions like institutions. In attacking the daunting problems posed by the AIDS epidemic, we bring our own background, resources, and values. It should not be surprising, then, that the world's oldest method of conflict resolution—politics—is often employed to reconcile our differences. This has been true throughout the epidemic, and was certainly true—and magnified—in the planning of the Sixth International Conference on AIDS. I have tried to use this magnification to focus a lens on the politics of AIDS as we enter the second decade of the most tragic health crisis of modern times.

As we organized the conference, I discovered intrigue, power plays, outsized egos, even humor. I sometimes was struck by the baseness of the maneuvering. At times, we might as well have been organizing a conference about speedboats, microcomputers, or selecting a Presidential nominee. Where was the concern about dying patients during the political machinations over travel restrictions, boycotts, and plenary invitations? In fact, the concern was omnipresent, energizing each battle with an urgency unique to this world conference. In his welcoming remarks to our conference delegates, Julius Krevans, Chancellor of the University of California, San Francisco, recalled a discreet sign he had once seen in a Chicago antique store. It read: THESE ITEMS ARE NOT VALUABLE BECAUSE THEY ARE OLD, THEY ARE OLD BECAUSE THEY ARE VALUABLE. "And so it is with AIDS," concluded Krevans. "It is not important because it is political, it is political because it is important."

The scientists, activists, politicians, and journalists I met while planning the conference were, almost without exception, good people trying to operate in a complex and constrained world. Most shared the same goal—to end the suffering wrought by AIDS. There were few white hats or black hats. Even within the groups we label with our preconceptions, I learned of markedly divergent goals, tactics, and agendas. Not all activists or all scientists think alike. Certainly not all HIV-infected people do.

Part of the story here is of my own growth. When I began working on the conference, I thought that I understood the world of AIDS. Since 1981, I had cared for hundreds of patients—watching in numbing frustration as the disease sapped weight, breath, spirit, and ultimately life from my patients and my friends. I had also studied and written at length about heart-wrenching ethical dilemmas, such as decisions about whether to use life-sustaining treatments—decisions confronted by all AIDS patients, their loved ones, and their doctors.

Once my work on the conference began, however, I quickly

recognized that I was a novice—totally unschooled in the politics of the epidemic. When I was called upon to enter the political arena—sometimes to advocate for what was right and sometimes to advocate for what was expedient—I often hesitated, not through lack of interest or commitment, but for fear of falling flat on my face.

My evolution over the eighteen months of planning the conference exemplifies, I think, the political evolution of the physician-scientist in the AIDS era. It is no longer acceptable —not in AIDS, at least—to ask patients to stand on the sidelines while doctors and researchers go about their work undisturbed. The empowerment of patients and the questioning of scientific expertise will be part of the sociological landscape of the 1990s—and not only in AIDS. Having our patients or our research subjects ask—or demand—to have an active voice in what we do and how we do it may be challenging, time-consuming, and even unpleasant. It is also undeniably right.

My goal in writing this book is to describe more than prescribe; to recount the planning of the Sixth International Conference on AIDS in a manner that illuminates the thinking of both the scientists and the activists racing to solve a problem of increasing complexity and outright horror. Perhaps the book will serve as a primer for both groups—to illustrate what they did wrong . . . and right.

But I would be dishonest if I claimed to be an impartial observer. My job was to advance and protect the vitality and very existence of the conference above all else, and this no doubt colored my outlook and actions. Whether my colleagues and I did our jobs well is left for others to judge. Like the epidemic itself, there were moments of disarray and defeat. But there were other moments—beautiful moments —in which activists and scientists marched side-by-side; moments in which researchers shed tears of grief and compassion after coming to understand, in an instant of clarity, what all of the anger is about. These moments convinced me of the power in the union of scientists and people living with AIDS. The coalition is fragile, but precious. With it, there is hope.

R.M.W.

OCTOBER 1990

THE PARABLE

God and a rabbi are discussing heaven and hell. "I will show you hell," said God, and they went into a room that had a large pot of stew in the middle. The smell was delicious, but around the pot sat people who were famished and desperate. All were holding spoons with very long handles that reached to the pot, but because the handles of the spoons were longer than their arms, it was impossible to get the stew back in their mouths. Their suffering was terrible.

"Now I will show you heaven," said God, and they went into an identical room. There was a similar pot of stew, and the people had identical spoons, but in this room they were well-nourished and happy, talking with each other.

At first the rabbi did not understand. "It is simple," said God. "You see, these people have learned to feed each other."

1 THE SQUASH GAME

S quash is a dangerous game. The contestants dart around a cube measuring 19 by 16 by 32 feet, bouncing off walls and each other. The hard rubber ball begins each match as an inert stone, but with continuous pounding takes on an elasticity and liveliness that make its itinerary increasingly unpredictable. The expert player understands this and learns to adapt to the changing speed and angle of his target; the novice is often left to stare blankly in sweaty frustration after swinging at thin air—at where the ball was *supposed* to be. So hazardous is squash that every squash racquet comes with its own disclaimer printed on its handle: "Due to the nature of the game of squash, equipment cannot be guaranteed."

I finished my squash match, and puffed my way toward the exit at the gymnasium at the University of California, San Francisco (UCSF). Although I had lost the game, the rest of my life was going smoothly in November 1988. I was a Robert Wood Johnson Clinical Scholar at Stanford University, pursuing my research interests in health policy and medical ethics. The work required time for quiet reflection, and life at Stanford was interesting, leisurely, and idyllic (a common Stanford triad); if I had any disquietude about my professional development, it was the lack of "real-world" experience. I briefly toyed with a stint in Washington, D.C., working as a Congressional underling, but rejected it as too ambitious and unpredictable. I plowed on with my fellowship, a somewhat removed but productive existence thinking and writing about life-sustaining treatments in AIDS.

Six months earlier, I had completed my chief residency in internal medicine at UCSF, a job often touted as a stepping-stone to academic greatness but one that provides its most rigorous training in fixing broken slide projectors and procuring quality donuts for hungry interns. During my chief residency, I continued to see cases of the disease that had, in many ways, dominated my medical training in the mid-1980s.

Actually, I had seen my first case of AIDS in 1982, a year before I moved to San Francisco, while a third-year medical student at the University of Pennsylvania in Philadelphia. My team had admitted to the hospital a young gay man with a bizarre history of progressive wasting, high spiking fevers, shortness of breath, and an atypical infiltrate on chest X ray. My attending physician, a sage internist named David Goldmann, had recently read reports of a strange new syndrome and quickly recognized our patient's case as fitting the syndrome's description. "This *thing*," he said—the syndrome had not yet been named—"will change the way we practice medicine."

There were doubters. After medical science's successes in understanding and conquering new diseases in the 1970s— Legionnaires' disease and toxic shock syndrome come to mind—it was easy to believe that AIDS too would be a short-lived distraction. Now, however, half a dozen years later, our initial innocence would have been almost comical had it not been so tragic. AIDS had proved a mighty foe; its toll was now measured by a body count in the tens of thousands. And there was no sign of salvation.

Caring for AIDS patients in the early years of the epidemic triggered a jumble of emotions: anguish, distaste, fear, challenge, excitement. The anguish came from watching people in the prime of their lives die tortured deaths, deaths that often seemed preferable to the preceding weeks of enfeeblement and breathlessness. The distaste stemmed from the lifestyles of the earliest gay AIDS patients, many of whom had averaged hundreds of anonymous and acrobatic sexual contacts yearly during the no-holds-barred 1970s. I had never viewed myself as homophobic, but I found my sensibilities tested each time I elicited a sexual history. The fear: In the early years, the agent responsible for AIDS and the routes of transmission had not yet been identified. My colleagues and I panicked each time we developed a cough, fever, or rash, wondering whether we might soon suffer the terrible fate of our patients.

But there was also a sense of challenge and excitement. In 1983, we began to realize—long before the *New York Times* and the White House—that we were living in a remarkable time and place. AIDS, it was clear, would challenge our most fundamental assumptions about the science and politics of health care: how it is organized, delivered, financed, and researched. To be part of it in San Francisco was to be surrounded by opportunity. Opportunity to help answer vital clinical and research questions, opportunity to help shape the future of medicine.

My own research efforts had resulted in several articles dealing with the use of the intensive care unit for patients with AIDS, one coauthored by a UCSF professor named Paul Volberding. Volberding, who at age forty was nine years my senior, had begun his faculty career as a young cancer specialist at San Francisco General Hospital when he was thirty-one. In *And the Band Played On*, Randy Shilts tells of Volberding's first patient after joining the faculty at San Francisco General. "There's the next great disease waiting for you," a senior oncologist had told him as he entered the room to examine a young man with Kaposi's sarcoma. KS, a virtually unknown skin tumor then, was something that he would see with tragic frequency over the remarkable decade that followed. Volberding was bright, energetic, and politically savvy. He quickly rose to become one of the world's best-known AIDS doctors; San Francisco's Mother Teresa, a local newspaper once called him.

Volberding was sitting by the gymnasium pool teaching his young son to swim as I left the squash court. He looked up as I walked by. "Boy, I really need to talk to you," he said. "Why don't you call me on Monday, and let's make plans for lunch."

The world of academic medicine being a far cry from Wall Street, the offer sounded a bit out of the ordinary. However, it wasn't until I returned home that evening and found a message on my answering machine from Dr. John Ziegler, the chairman of UCSF's AIDS task force and a professor at the Veteran's Hospital in San Francisco, that I knew something was brewing. Ziegler mentioned that there was a project he and Volberding were working on and they might need my help. Again, let's do lunch.

We met four days later. "I'm not sure if you know anything about the International Conference on AIDS," Ziegler began. I knew a bit, having attended the 1986 conference in Paris to present a paper. "In June 1990, the conference will be in San Francisco. Paul and I are the cochairs, and we'd like to show you the organization we envision for the conference."

Ziegler, whose years as an administrator at the National Cancer Institute made him a whiz at organizational charts, began drawing lines and boxes on the blackboard, which quickly took on the appearance of an octopus. Policy would be decided upon by a local organizing committee, composed of UCSF's top AIDS scientists and clinicians. The most important part of the organization, Ziegler continued, was the Program Committee. "The conference has gravitated toward social issues in the past few years," he said. "We really want to put on a scientific conference." The Program Committee was divided into four thematic tracks—basic science, clinical science and trials, epidemiology and prevention, and social science and policy. The latter track—dubbed Track D—had only been added recently; the initial plans were to have a separate policy conference outside the main gathering, so as to emphasize to the maximum the scientific aspects of AIDS research.

Oh, so this is what they are getting at, I thought. They want me to be a member of the Track D committee. But these are two very busy men—they can't possibly spend this much time recruiting each of the dozens of members of the track committees. Another thought dawned on me. Maybe they want me to *chair* the Track D committee! I began to sweat at the size of the responsibility. Ziegler continued drawing tentacles.

"In the middle of all this will be a program director," Ziegler said. "This person will supervise the entire organization: the four program tracks, a communications committee, a fundraising committee, an international visitors committee, and a large press and community-relations contingent. He'll be working in an incredibly delicate political environment and supervising a budget of six or seven million dollars." I wondered who they had in mind. If I chaired Track D, I'd be working closely with this person. Ziegler drew a circle in the middle of the octopus to highlight the central position of the Program Director, and turned to me and smiled. "We want you for this job," he said.

The decision by Ziegler and Volberding to offer me the position was, in part, a flattering commentary on my clinical and research activities during my years of medical training. But the decision was also motivated by my potential availability: The chairmen realized that the jobs of planning the program and helping to coordinate the administrative and political aspects of the conference required a full-time commitment for eighteen months. More senior physician-researchers, entrenched in existing responsibilities, would be unable or unwilling to provide the requisite time.

But, in accepting the position, I worried that I too would pay a price. I would forgo patient care and teaching for more than a year. My skills would suffer, and I would miss these, my two most satisfying professional activities, profoundly. Academically, I worried that interrupting my research for an extended period would place me well behind my peers in the quest for a desirable faculty position. Finally, I worried that the conference—which seemed to grow more politically volatile each year—could prove a divisive fiasco, forever branding me as navigator of the Titanic of the AIDS epidemic.

On the other hand, I was intrigued by the opportunity. The challenge of trying to forge a vibrant and meaningful event was nearly irresistible. I would be helping to shape the worldwide clinical, research, and policy agenda in AIDS for the 1990s. And, more practically, the personal contacts I would make and the visibility I would enjoy could not possibly hurt my career . . . unless things went badly.

In the end, I accepted the job of Program Director, but only after locking in a UCSF faculty position to begin after the conference, no matter what. As Ronald Reagan loved to say of his arms negotiations with the Soviets: Trust but verify.

Over the course of the month-long discussions that preceded my acceptance, I came to better understand the conference and my role. I began to appreciate the organizational complexities involved, and the logistical nightmare of planning a meeting for twelve thousand participants and two thousand members of the international press. I also gained a better sense of the politics of AIDS, and realized that this would add somewhat to the challenge.

But it wasn't until the meeting of the International Steering Committee of the Fifth International Conference on AIDS in Montreal in February 1989 that I fully appreciated the rarified air I was going to breathe. Barely two weeks into my tenure as Program Director of the Sixth International Conference on AIDS, the Montreal organizers called and asked if we wanted to send a representative to their planning meeting. Since at that moment I presided over a staff of one—me—I seemed like the logical person to go.

I entered the conference room in Montreal's Meridien Hotel and found a who's who of international AIDS dignitaries. Seated at the table were Dr. Jonathan Mann, head of the World Health Organization's AIDS program, Dr. Lars Olof Kallings, President of the International AIDS Society, and Ivan Head, former Canadian Prime Minister Pierre Trudeau's top advisor and now chairman of the Montreal meeting. Also present was Dr. Richard Morisset, Montreal's Program Director. Morisset, a venerable Montreal clinician, was at least fifteen years my senior—I had felt young before I arrived in Montreal, but now I felt like I was in junior high school. How exactly did I end up in this company, I thought. I resolved to speak only when spoken to; that way they wouldn't brand me an imposter.

The Montreal conference was four months away, and the principals discussed the mushrooming budget. I frantically scribbled notes. The conversation then turned to the question of whether to invite Dr. C. Everett Koop, the renowned Surgeon General of the United States, to participate in the conference program. Mann, Kallings, and Head turned toward me, the only American resident at the table. "Bob," Ivan Head asked, "how will Dr. Koop feel if we don't invite him?" My relationship with Dr. Koop was not exactly intimate at that point: I'd once seen him lecture from about fifty rows back as a medical student in Philadelphia. "I don't think he'll have a problem with it," I answered, shaking my head knowingly. "Fine," said Head, and the discussion moved on.

I allowed myself a tinge of pride for this, my first baby step on the road to leadership. The ball had come to me, and I had struck it squarely and aggressively. But it was far too early to be cocky, for the ball was still cool, its bounces predictable.

2 MONTREAL, JUNE 1989

Helicopters whirred above Montreal's convention center, challenging the monotony of the slate-gray sky. The day was Sunday, June 4, 1989; the Fifth International Conference on AIDS would begin in an hour. The helicopters doubtless represented security for the Prime Minister of Canada and the President of Zambia, who would soon address the conference's opening ceremony. Despite the traditional turgidity of such ceremonies—in which dignitaries intone inspiring words about the epidemic and their indispensable role in combatting it—my interest was genuine. The events of the day would be highly instructive for my planning. As I walked toward the convention center, my strides grew faster and more rhythmic, mirroring the revolutions of the choppers' blades. I joined the sea of delegates pushing past lethargic security guards as we entered the hall.

The delegates came from 130 nations, each nation changed irrevocably by the decade of AIDS. Perhaps the coming decade would bring better news. Perhaps this conference would reveal the eagerly awaited breakthrough. Perhaps.

Ten minutes before the ceremony was to begin, we heard a commotion in the back of the huge hall. Two hundred and fifty young men and women wearing T-shirts and carrying placards swept past the helpless security personnel and mounted the stage. "They say *get* back, we say *fight* back!" they chanted. "AIDS action now!" Although I had attended a few of the Montreal planning meetings and been in close contact with the organizers, I hadn't heard about any plans for a demonstration before the conference opening. Still, I naively wondered whether this had been preplanned. I made a mental note to ask the organizers about that. In any case, the demonstration made good theater; it would make a lively opening salvo on tomorrow's network news. The scientists and physicians in the audience, generally supportive of the activists' chants for more funding and less discrimination, cheered and clapped. And then they waited. And waited.

Scientist talked with scientist, physician with physician as everyone waited for the protest to end and the conference to begin. The mood remained upbeat and anticipatory. This protest will end soon, many thought, as they took advantage of the unplanned break to catch up on the latest AIDS news and gossip with their colleagues in the audience.

Twenty minutes after taking the stage, one of the Canadian protestors grabbed the center-stage mike. I wondered if it was turned on. It was. "On behalf of people with AIDS," he boomed, "I would like to officially open the Fifth International Conference on AIDS." Decrying the AIDS policy of Canadian Prime Minister Brian Mulroney, who was sequestered backstage, the activist, emboldened by the size of his audience, continued: "This conference will change international AIDS conferences forever!" I cringed.

The audience waited patiently as the group's spokesman began to walk off the stage with most of the protestors. However, forty members of the group remained and began exhorting the rest to stay. "Read the manifesto," many chanted. It was obvious that splinter groups had formed and the putative leader of the activists had lost control. Claude Paul Boivin, the Executive Director of the Montreal conference, bravely took the stage and pleaded, "I ask you to respect the arrangement." As it developed, the "arrangement" had been hastily negotiated as the protestors stormed the front gates and phalanxes of activists rushed past unprepared guards into the main hall. Boivin and the other conference organizers had met with a few of the protestors and agreed to activate the stage microphone for ten minutes in exchange for the protestors' leaving the hall at the end of their demonstration. But a number of the protestors were not ready to keep their side of the bargain. After fifteen more minutes on stage, many took seats in the conspicuous block of three hundred empty chairs front and center, the reserved VIP section. "We're the VIPs," shouted the activists.

Although I had heard of the AIDS activist groups and had some concerns that they might target the San Francisco conference, I blithely assumed that they and the scientists shared a common enemy: the AIDS virus. Why would the activists, whose hopes for cures and vaccines rode squarely on the shoulders of the scientists, attack a scientific conference, I asked myself. That question would be asked of me in a hundred ways a hundred times during the next year. A close look at the faces of players in the ongoing drama of the opening ceremony in Montreal provided some insight. The protestors, who were mostly from ACT UP (the AIDS Coalition to Unleash Power), looked like central casting for protestors of the Sixties—young, exhilarated, furious, and intoxicated by their own power. The scientists and doctors sitting in the audience, older and more conservative, had mildly curious looks on their faces that would soon turn to boredom, and then to anger and impatience as the shouting wore on.

The Montreal organizers met frantically to develop a strategy to deal with this unexpected disruption. Wanting to avoid a confrontation at all costs, they decided to begin the conference only after the protestors left the hall. Consequently, the audience sat for ninety minutes waiting for movement.

Dr. Jonathan Mann, Director of the Global Programme on AIDS (GPA) of the World Health Organization, left his seat to join the negotiations. Mann, who in his three years at GPA had built the organization into the world's most important international AIDS agency, was highly respected by the activists as well as the scientists.

Mann spoke to the protestors and helped negotiate a settlement. The activists were allowed to remain in the hall, and they were relatively quiet during the course of the ceremony —that is, until Prime Minister Mulroney's address, which was greeted by renewed catcalls, hisses, and boos from the few dozen protestors remaining in the auditorium.

Kenneth Kaunda, President of Zambia, saved what could be saved of the opening program. In a stirring address, Kaunda spoke eloquently about the developed world's diversion of resources to building nuclear weapons when such resources could be used to stem the destruction of the AIDS virus. He called AIDS "a silent nuclear bomb, which kills with no explosion but is just as devastating." The President's loss of a son to AIDS a few years earlier gave his remarks a special poignancy. Kaunda had planned to say much more about the importance of global solidarity in fighting the epidemic, but was forced to cut his speech short because of the activists' delays.

The tanks of the Chinese Army rolled into Tienanmen Square and the Ayatollah Khomeini died during the first two days of the Montreal conference. That these events pushed the International AIDS Conference off the front pages of many newspapers may have been a blessing. Much of the news coverage of the conference emphasized the protests and what many saw as the "circus atmosphere" of the meeting.

The activism extended beyond the opening ceremony. When Stephen Joseph, New York City's Commissioner of Health, rose to speak, a crowd of ACT UPers began yelling, "Resign! Resign! Resign!" The activists then turned their backs on Dr. Joseph, screaming, "Murder!" and "Shame!" throughout the rest of his speech. At the opening ceremony, many scientists in the audience had been simply bored waiting for the session to begin. Today, they were livid. Had they been asked, many would have agreed with the activists that throughout the epidemic New York City had woefully underfunded its AIDS effort and ignored prevention and treatment programs that could have saved hundreds, perhaps thousands of lives. As the shouting persisted, however, the audience became more impressed by Dr. Joseph's courage in persevering with his talk than they were with the activists and their message. When the Health Commissioner finished speaking, the audience gave him a standing ovation.

The noon press conference was just as unpleasant. Three hundred members of the international press attended, and plenary speakers were available to answer questions on a wide range of international issues, including prevention efforts among Thai schoolchildren and prostitutes. However, virtually every question was directed at Dr. Joseph and dealt with parochial New York AIDS politics. Most of the questioners were not journalists, but New York activists who had bullied their way into the press briefing room. And later that day, when Dr. Ellen Cooper of the Food and Drug Administration finished her talk on the drug approval process, an activist rushed to a microphone and screamed, "You're a murderer! You're the Mafia who plays God!"

The audience of scientists and clinicians was shocked. Many had attended contentious and controversial lectures in their careers, and had heard presentations met with probing and even derisive questions and comments from the audience. But this? Many did not pause to consider whether the activists' points were valid, so incensed were they over the abrasive tactics.

While some scientists and journalists spoke of the damage done to the meeting by the protests, others focussed on the street theater. Many remarked that the conference had degenerated into an "AIDS convention." The point was made graphically just outside the convention center, where a hot air balloon in the shape of a condom rose 120 feet above the onlookers. For reporters needing to plan their day, the sign in the press room advertised NEXT ERECTION: 2 P.M. Meanwhile, four prostitutes sauntered past a stunned crowd in the exhibition hall, shouting, "Get it while it's hot, boys!" and then naming their prices for the performance of various sex acts. Their appearance, they said, was designed to demonstrate that too much blame for heterosexual transmission of the human immunodeficiency virus (HIV, the causative agent of AIDS) had been placed on them, and not enough on their clients.

Some important science was presented at the Montreal conference. The advent of new therapies led to cautious optimism among patients and caregivers. Two such therapies were zidovudine (also known as AZT), which slows the replication of HIV, and aerosolized pentamidine, which markedly decreases the incidence of *Pneumocystis carinii* pneumonia, the most common and deadly opportunistic infection in AIDS. For the first time, many spoke of AIDS as a "manageable chronic disease." The analogy was made to insulin injections, which do not cure diabetes but forestall its life-threatening manifestations for many decades. The same hope was expressed for the management of HIV infection.

Despite the encouraging news about treatments, the epidemiologic reports were bleak. Only a few years earlier, forecasters speculated that one in ten people with HIV infection would eventually develop clinical disease and die of AIDS; the predictions now were that at least two in three would die. Each year, at conference after conference, the predictions seemed to grow more pessimistic. The true risk that a person with HIV infection would die of AIDS might eventually prove to be 100 percent.

Researchers studying the impoverished developing coun-

tries of the world arrived with more grim news. Dr. Jonathan
Mann of the World Health Organization pegged the number
of HIV-infected people worldwide at five to ten million. Paint-
ing a picture of extraordinary death and suffering in years to
come, Mann spoke of a ten- to twentyfold rise in the rate of
infection among intravenous drug users and prostitutes in
Thailand. Similar increases were reported for risk groups in
cities in West Africa and Brazil.

Despite the importance of the scientific information, the
critical story of Montreal was the unfolding conflict between
scientists and activists. Randy Shilts, whose book *And the
Band Played On* was the first detailed analysis of the politics
of the AIDS epidemic, proclaimed that the conference ushered
in an "era of bad feelings." Reviewing the conference for
Mother Jones magazine, Shilts wrote, "By the end of this
year's Montreal conference, AIDS activists and scientists
hated each other even more than before. If you were HIV-
positive, would you feel better?" And at his speech at the
closing ceremony of the conference, Shilts scolded the activists. "Expressing anger can give you a warm, fuzzy feeling
inside," he told the audience, "but this conference is not
supposed to be a therapy session . . . It is not enough to be
angry, if that anger is not paired with intelligence about its
best tactical timing and its best strategic targets." For this,
he too was heckled by some in the crowd.

Many of the scientists at Montreal spoke of avoiding future
conferences. Some even considered leaving AIDS work altogether. One prominent AIDS clinician, a cancer specialist by
training, shook his head after a particularly unpleasant session. "I kind of enjoy treating women with breast cancer.
Maybe that's what I should be doing. It would be a hell of
a lot easier than this."

But most of the comments were directed at the conference
itself. Dr. Robert Gallo of the U.S. National Cancer Institute
felt that "the scientific aspects of the conference had not been
given adequate representation." He was asked whether he

and other researchers would attend next year's San Francisco conference. "Some basic scientists will, and some basic scientists won't," was his reply. "Scientists need the time and the quiet to reflect."

Dr. Luc Montagnier of the Pasteur Institute in Paris, generally credited with the discovery of HIV, echoed similar thoughts. "On the one hand, I can understand the need for scientists to be in contact with the patients. What I understand less is that they make intrusions in the scientific meetings."

And Dr. William Blattner, Editor of the *Journal of AIDS*, wrote: "Unless AIDS meetings evolve into a more productive format, the utility of such meetings for scientific exchange will be lost and top scientists will seek other smaller and more cordial environments to share data critical to solving this problem. Future meetings at best will be characterized by token appearances by top scientists because of the hassles, disruptions, and other problems which characterized the Montreal meeting. One can only hope that there is still time to reform the format and transform this meeting of international importance into a productive venue for promoting a solution to the pandemic of AIDS."

3 GENEALOGY OF A CONFERENCE

The challenges we faced in organizing the 1990 meeting are placed in sharp relief not only by Montreal, but by an examination of the history of all the International Conferences on AIDS.

THE ATLANTA CONFERENCE

The First International Conference on AIDS, at the Centers for Disease Control in Atlanta in 1985, was a largely scientific affair. Although the audience of two thousand contained a smattering of gay activists, the bulk of the participants were researchers presenting and listening to data about this latter-day plague. Since the first reports of a strange disease killing gay men in San Francisco, New York, and Los Angeles in 1981, there had been about ten thousand cases of AIDS and five thousand deaths by the time of the Atlanta conference. The mood at the conference, as audiences listened to four hundred oral and poster research presentations, was one of shock, despite the discovery of the causative agent one year earlier and the development of effective screening tests for HIV. It was now clear that the problem of AIDS was not going to be solved quickly, as toxic shock syndrome and Legionnaires' disease had been in the 1970s. The body count, which was doubling yearly, was expected to do so for the foreseeable future. And the worldwide effects of AIDS on public health and health policy would be staggering.

Although people with AIDS and their advocates did not make their presence strongly felt in Atlanta, the meeting, like all aspects of the epidemic, had a political side. U.S. Secretary of Health and Human Services Margaret Heckler, in an address at the opening ceremony of the conference, promised that "AIDS will remain our number-one public health priority until it has been conquered." This, despite the fact that the word "AIDS" had not been uttered publicly by the American President, and the level of funding for research and education ($93 million in 1985) was woefully inadequate considering the gravity of the problem. Many observers of the federal effort felt that the government would not take AIDS seriously until it attacked heterosexuals or movie stars (in the end, it took both to turn the tide), and their suspicions were not allayed by Heckler's comments. "We must conquer AIDS before it affects the heterosexual population and the general population," she said. "We have a very strong public interest in stopping AIDS before it spreads outside the risk groups, before it becomes an overwhelming problem."

THE PARIS CONFERENCE

By the time of the 1986 conference in Paris, world attention had been riveted on the exploding epidemic by the death of Rock Hudson. The intensity of the media coverage meant that the research presented at the conference no longer induced shock. Instead, a sense of unmitigated pessimism enveloped the convention center like a shroud. It was now clear that HIV did not simply enjoy attacking immune cells; it also thrived on the cells of the central nervous system, often leading to disabling dementia. But that was only part of the problem. It was now also possible that HIV would find the brain to be a sanctuary, protected from the effects of otherwise effective antiviral agents behind the relatively impermeable "blood-brain barrier." Some researchers raised the horrifying specter of large numbers of young, demented AIDS patients whose cognitive functions degenerated steadily despite being cured of their systemic infection by effective antivirals.

People also despaired at the news from the developing world. AIDS had now been identified as the cause of the deadly syndrome of diarrhea and wasting that was taking tens of thousands of lives in sub-Saharan Africa. Dubbed "slim disease" by the Africans, Third World researchers feared a much greater obstacle to the dissemination of effective therapies than the blood-brain barrier: namely, money. The average health care expenditure of many of the countries devastated by AIDS in Africa was less than one dollar per person per year. Hundreds of thousands would die a tormented death without any hope of treatment.

With the recognition that AIDS was an international problem without immediate solution, the top AIDS researchers and clinicians identified the need for an international society. Such a society could help coordinate the global response to the epidemic, set policies, and support an ongoing series of international meetings. It was clear that the International Conferences on AIDS were a critical part of the worldwide effort to fight AIDS, an indispensable forum for the dissemination of new scientific information. In the Paris conference's atmosphere of despair, the International AIDS Society (IAS) was conceived, and the seeds of the next six yearly international conferences were planted. As often happens in such endeavors, the location of the meetings was highly correlated with the hometowns of the original IAS members. The Third Conference would be in Washington, D.C.; its chair was IAS board member George Galasso of the National Institutes of Health. The Fourth International Conference would be held in Stockholm, Sweden, not coincidentally the home of IAS

President Lars Olof Kallings. Paul Volberding and Jay Levy of UCSF lobbied to bring 1989's Fifth Conference to San Francisco. However, the planning meeting was hosted by a group from Montreal, led by IAS board member Alastair Clayton, the director of Canada's Federal Centre for AIDS. So the Fifth Conference went to Montreal, with a San Francisco conference to follow a year later. Thus, in 1990, San Francisco would become the first city at the epicenter of the epidemic to host an International Conference on AIDS.

THE WASHINGTON CONFERENCE

The events of 1986 and early 1987 guaranteed extensive interest in the Third International Conference on AIDS. Surgeon General C. Everett Koop's report on AIDS was a sensation, shocking his conservative backers by bluntly calling for widespread AIDS education and explicit prevention efforts. Koop's report, coming on the heels of the death of Rock Hudson, gave AIDS a new legitimacy, and Koop immediately became a media superstar. Press interest reached record levels: 850 registered journalists descended on the Washington meeting. Although the organizers at the National Institutes of Health anticipated an audience of about 3,500, more than 6,000 registrants packed the halls of the Washington Hilton. The amount of research presented at the meeting also exploded: Nearly 2,000 papers were submitted for review, and about two-thirds of these were presented.

In addition to the growth of the scientific aspects of the meeting, the location of the Third Conference on AIDS in the nation's capital lent an unavoidable political cast to the proceedings. President Ronald Reagan bowed to public pressure to deliver his first speech on the epidemic at a gala event on the eve of the conference. By the time of his speech, more than twenty thousand Americans were dead of AIDS. The keynote address at the opening ceremony of the conference was given by George Bush, then Vice President.

Just as the presence of the President and Vice President demonstrated their recognition of the importance of the AIDS conference as a political event, members of the increasingly sophisticated and politicized gay community were beginning to recognize the same thing. Bush and Reagan were intermittently heckled during their speeches. However, most of the activists were congregated outside the convention hall and around the White House. On the nightly news broadcasts, the world saw pictures of demonstrators being arrested by police wearing bright yellow, arm-length gloves. Although research had by now proved that the AIDS virus could not be passed through casual contact, the sight of the gloves served to reinforce the public's general overestimation of the risk of HIV transmission.

THE STOCKHOLM CONFERENCE

By the time planning for the 1990 conference really got underway in January 1989, many AIDS researchers were already looking back fondly on the Fourth International Conference, held in Stockholm in 1988. Much of the praise was directed at the ample meeting space, the superb social events, and the quality of the scientific presentations—and after the Montreal meeting, many people happily recalled the absence of activism at the Stockholm conference. Stockholm had been a chance to do some "real science." The perspective of AIDS sufferers was compressed into a program of lectures and videos called "The Face of AIDS," which played each day during lunch hour. Some HIV-infected people would later complain that, by separating the sessions dealing with their concerns from those of the main conference agenda, they had been "marginalized." But many scientists commented favorably on the format, having been spared the shrill and desperate cries of those affected by the disease they dispassionately studied.

* * *

The first five International Conferences on AIDS reflected an increasing number of fundamental issues being played out in the newly built arena of AIDS politics. The conflict between scientists and activists that reached a head in Montreal represented a fractious attempt to answer the question: Whose conference (and whose epidemic) is this, anyway? With the passing of each year came increased world interest in the conference. This meant that all the players had more to gain from pursuing their own agendas at the yearly meeting.

THE SCIENTISTS

The scientists and clinicians at the international conferences felt they had the most to lose, since it was "their" conference to begin with. The goals of the researchers and clinicians attending the conference vary. Many attend to learn the state of the art in their own fields of study, which helps them in their work. Others, including doctors, nurses, dentists, social workers, and psychologists, come to hear about other disciplines that complement their area of primary interest. Still others go to network. The conference provides a rare opportunity for an epidemiologist from San Francisco to meet a virologist from Bethesda, a clinician from Hong Kong, and a public health worker from Kinshasa. These interactions are always interesting, and often result in meaningful collaborations.

Many researchers attend the international conferences to present their own work. Not only are all scientists gratified when the fruits of their research are used by others, but such presentations help researchers gain academic prestige and promotion.

Finally, the public's commonly held view of medical conferences, in which scientists or clinicians hear a presentation or two in the morning before donning their golf attire, has some basis in fact. This probably takes place less at the International Conference on AIDS than at, say, a conference on "Marketing Your Medical Practice" at a Caribbean hotel, but it certainly motivates some to attend the meeting.

Noticeably absent from the wish-list of most scientists attending the international conferences are two other goals: furthering a political agenda and appreciating the perspective of persons with the disease being discussed. One does not expect to hear someone heckle a government speaker for not adequately funding arthritis research at a rheumatology conference. And an emphysema conference in which wheezing patients sit next to scientists—unthinkable. Yet many scientists at the Montreal meeting saw the AIDS conference moving in this direction. In fact, this movement was inevitable, driven by the other major players, whose goals were far different from those of the scientists.

ACTIVISTS AND PEOPLE WITH AIDS

HIV-infected people have living within them time bombs that will at some unpredictable moment destroy their immune systems and lead to their deaths. That many of these people take an intense interest in treatment options for their condition should not surprise. Perhaps we should be more surprised that patients with other diseases lack the same intensity of interest. In any case, increasing numbers of people with AIDS (commonly called PWAs) attend the international conferences on AIDS to learn of new therapies to treat themselves or loved ones.

It is important to distinguish between activists and the HIV-infected communities. Not every AIDS activist is HIV-infected, and certainly not every HIV-infected person is an activist. Some of the people angriest at the demonstrators in Montreal were nonactivist PWAs, who worried audibly about alienating the scientists. Nevertheless, the activists on stage at the opening ceremony in Montreal recognized a media opportunity when they saw one. With the world's attention focussed on AIDS for the week, what better chance to shape the political agenda than to demonstrate?

The political agenda of the activists in recent years has been to expedite the development of new drugs for AIDS. To many activists, politicians inadequately fund drug research, scientists develop and test drugs too slowly (and are often working on the wrong drugs even if the pace is adequate), regulators approve new medications too sluggishly, and pharmaceutical companies price drugs too expensively. Although most American AIDS activists are gay men, the activist community has agitated over AIDS in women, AIDS in minority populations, and even AIDS in the developing world. But when push comes to shove, the activists' agenda usually reverts closer to home: finding new drugs to prolong the lives of the HIV-infected. And the activists' successes in this arena—expediting the testing and approval of drugs for life-threatening pneumonias, sight-threatening eye infections, and HIV itself—are incontrovertible.

But even these successes have a dark connotation for many activists. In recent years, research alleging a slowing in the pace of the epidemic has been met with howls of protest from activists who claim such findings will provide unsympathetic policymakers an excuse to slash funding for AIDS. Similarly, the mantra that AIDS is turning into a "manageable chronic disease" is often met with fear and hostility. Lawrence Gostin, Executive Director of the American Society of Law and Medicine, echoes the sentiments of many activists. "The costs of perceiving AIDS as a chronic disease are considerable and should be resisted," wrote Gostin. "If AIDS is viewed as a chronic disease, it could sink to the mediocre level of health policy, research, and financing to which other chronic diseases have been relegated."

THE MEDIA

The media has rightly been criticized for ignoring AIDS until well after the epidemic had claimed thousands of lives. The usual explanation—that the afflicted were from disenfranchised groups in society: gays and minority drug users—is too facile. However, it certainly is a large part of the explanation. Just consider the press coverage AIDS would have received had it struck stockbrokers on Wall Street or Midwestern farmers with the same viciousness. But there is more. The AIDS story is intellectually complex and challenging to cover. All this talk of seropositivity, T-helper and suppressor counts, and exponential growth is not the stuff of evening news sound bites. The international conferences represent an opportunity for the media to concentrate its attention on AIDS for five days. All the appropriate and quotable individuals are in one place, and all the competition is there as well. So most news organizations find the conference irresistible.

The week of the conference is hellish for journalists. A few days before the Montreal meeting, reporters were handed the volume of abstracts (the size of the New York City telephone directory), and began diving for pearls amidst the 5,700 published reports. "The existence of the conference gives the stories a timeliness that they wouldn't otherwise have," Paul Raeburn of the Associated Press observed after his week of diving in Montreal. Many journalists found covering the Montreal conference particularly challenging, as they scrambled to report on both research presentations and activism. For the first time in the history of medical conferences, major newspapers and television stations would send both scientific and political correspondents to report on the San Francisco meeting.

THE POLITICIANS

Finally, where one finds media, one will usually find politicians. Politicians may use the conference to demonstrate instant "commitment" to the plight of PWAs. Although in the United States such evidence of commitment may raise the ire of the conservatives, a number of politicians have found it in their interest to be present. In fact, if President Reagan's appearance on the eve of the 1987 Washington conference is counted, the heads of the host government addressed each of the three conferences prior to San Francisco.

THE FRAGILE COALITION

Ivan Head, Chairman of the Montreal meeting, summed up the conference this way: "The Fifth International Conference on AIDS . . . drew together for the first time—not always harmoniously—the several groups that must participate in the quest for solutions. And it did so in a fully international way, involving many hundreds of scientists and experts from the developing countries; another first.

"The full involvement of behavioral and social scientists, the attention given to legal, ethical, economic, and political issues, the involvement of the pharmaceutical firms engaged in research, the presence of sometimes raucous activists— these elements confirmed in a lively yet overwhelmingly serious fashion that AIDS is not simply a laboratory issue . . ."

Head was correct. All of the conference's constituencies *do* need to participate in the quest for solutions. Although one might assume that each group shares an interest in finding such solutions, in Montreal it appeared that they shared little else. Despite their differences, these groups represent a coalition, albeit a fragile one, with immense power to effect changes in the fight against AIDS. But, we asked ourselves after Montreal, could the coalition be unified? Or would its divergent interests inexorably tear it apart?

This, then, represented our challenge in organizing the San Francisco conference. While each of the players pursued a parochial agenda, we would pursue ours: to bring together in a cooperative, collaborative way all of the diverse participants. We would need to act as AIDS mediators: to hear the concerns of each group and translate them to the others, so that the result would best serve the many. As I packed up to leave Montreal, I realized that the job before us might just be impossible. With all of these constituencies, each of them increasingly speaking of "us vs. them," how could our conference be anything but divisive and counterproductive?

Some members of the press have argued that there would be little lost if the International AIDS Conference collapsed under its own weight, like a tumor necrosing as it outgrows its blood supply. After all, the past few conferences provided few scientific "breakthroughs." In fact, one of the changes wrought by the AIDS epidemic has been an ethical consensus that deems it wrong to withhold potentially lifesaving results waiting for a conference or for publication. In keeping with this consensus, many of the breakthroughs in AIDS are revealed at press conferences or more specialized scientific caucuses, no longer awaiting the annual international meeting. What is really the value of such a gathering, especially given the time and resources expended in its planning?

I see the conference as having importance in four areas. First, a tremendous amount of information is disseminated, often leading to important collaborations and partnerships. When I presented my data on intensive care for people with AIDS to an audience of three hundred at the Montreal conference, I mentioned that I was interested in working with investigators at other sites. Researchers from New York, Los Angeles, Vancouver—even Oakland, only a bridge away from San Francisco—approached me to join what has proved to be an important collaboration. Had there been no conference, we never would have joined forces. This scenario plays out hundreds of times at every international AIDS conference.

Moreover, the information-sharing role of the conference is particularly crucial for the hundreds of delegates from the developing countries of the world. AIDS is a holocaust in countries like Uganda and Zaire; the conference provides caregivers and researchers from countries like these access to potentially lifesaving information, unobtainable from any other source.

Second, with so many problems competing for recognition,

the meeting provides a compelling—and photogenic—opportunity for the media to focus its powerful lens on AIDS. The conference guarantees that at least for five days each year AIDS will be a front-runner in the race for society's attention, attention that translates into needed resources from the public and private sectors.

Third, the chance for the participants—be they doctors, scientists, PWAs, or activists—to unite provides a necessary opportunity for renewal. Studies on "AIDS burnout" demonstrate clinical depression in about one-third of health care workers caring for large numbers of PWAs. The conference provides a much-needed opportunity to recharge the psychic batteries.

Finally, the conference is a milestone; a yearly pause to reflect on where we have been, where we are, and where we are going. It is a vital, if unwieldy, looking glass through which most of the forces shaping the epidemic may be observed and analyzed. And so the pages that follow are not simply a chronicle of the planning of a world AIDS conference. They tell the story of the forces shaping the global fight against AIDS. These forces hold in their hands the potential to save, or to lose, untold numbers of lives.

4 IMPRISONED IN MINNEAPOLIS

On April 2, 1989, Hans Paul Verhoef, a pleasant, soft-spoken thirty-one-year-old AIDS educator from Delft, Holland, left his native country to fly to San Francisco to attend the 11th National Gay and Lesbian Health Conference. Verhoef hoped to learn about American programs for dealing with AIDS. One American program he had not expected to learn about was the one whose cornerstone was the list of "dangerous and contagious diseases."

But Verhoef had AIDS. When his plane landed in Minneapolis for a brief stopover, he told the Immigration and Naturalization Services (INS) agent that he was heading for the San Francisco health conference. The official searched his bag and found Verhoef's supply of AZT, a letter he had written about travelling with AIDS, some sexual paraphernalia, and a gay guidebook. Under the provisions of Public Law 100-71, also known as the Helms amendment, passed by the Senate a year earlier, Verhoef was ineligible to enter the United States. And so began our predicament.

The story of the Helms amendment began a century before it was unwittingly challenged by Hans Paul Verhoef. In 1891, the Congress of the United States passed a law excluding, for the purposes of immigration, "idiots, insane persons, paupers . . . and persons suffering from a loathsome or contagious disease." The pejorative "loathsome" was dropped in 1961 and replaced by the general term "dangerous and contagious diseases." The intent of excluding individuals on this list of "dangerous and contagious diseases" is twofold: to prevent transmission of contagious diseases to American citizens, and to limit the use of American tax dollars on health care for aliens. On the face of it, the concept is laudable, albeit parochial.

Until 1987, the list included five venereal diseases (syphilis, gonorrhea, and three more obscure conditions: chancroid, lymphogranuloma venereum, and granuloma inguinale), infectious leprosy, and active tuberculosis. The task of compiling and updating the list traditionally fell to the Centers for Disease Control (CDC) in Atlanta. However, politics always being the dark shadow of science when it comes to AIDS, the Reagan Administration and the U.S. Senate entered the debate about the list in 1987. The decision to modify the list would later become one of the major policy challenges ever faced by the AIDS community and result in an international boycott of the Sixth International Conference on AIDS. But few could foresee the implications of the addition of HIV to the list in 1987. And so it went virtually unnoticed.

A casual observer might say, as did Senator Robert Dole of Kansas in the Senate debate on the matter, that "there is every reason to add the AIDS virus to this list, as there is no question regarding its being dangerous or contagious." Dangerous, no doubt. But the statement overlooks the exceptional resistance of HIV to spread by casual contact, the usual connotation of "contagious." Indeed, to acquire HIV infection from another requires the acquirer to engage in a known risky activity: unsafe sexual practices, needle-sharing, or (rarely) transfusion of infected blood products.

The addition of HIV to the list of "dangerous and contagious diseases" in 1987 resulted from a complex series of administrative and legislative activities that had begun a year earlier. Conservative Senator Jesse Helms of North Carolina is generally cast as the villain in latter-day recounting; however, a survey of the events at the time reveals others who bear responsibility as well.

The United States Public Health Service (PHS), which includes the CDC, as well as the National Institutes of Health (NIH) and the Food and Drug Administration (FDA), proposed amending its regulations to add AIDS to the list of dangerous contagious diseases in 1986. At first, PHS—concerned with possible discrimination against individuals in high-risk groups—recommended only that people with clinical AIDS be excluded (thus obviating the requirement for HIV testing of immigrants, who might harbor the virus but remain asymptomatic). In May 1987, however, the agency broadened its recommendation to exclude all immigrants with HIV infection. Throughout the deliberations, the CDC supported the concept of adding HIV to the dangerous disease list. President Reagan also indicated that he favored the addition.

The issue soon reached the floor of the Senate. On June 2, 1987, the Senate debated a bill to appropriate $30 million to supply AZT to needy AIDS patients. Senator Helms offered an amendment. "None of the funds appropriated by this Act for the emergency provision of drugs," read the amendment, "shall be expended after August 31, 1987, if on that date the President has not . . . added HIV infection to the list of dangerous contagious diseases."

Political pundit Hedrick Smith has described Helms's power as "porcupine power"—the power to be prickly; the ability and willingness to block important legislation to achieve one's goals. Senator Helms continued to lecture his fellow Senators.

He cited statistics on the worldwide explosion of HIV. He claimed (without substantiation) that the President had already directed the Secretary of Health and Human Services to add HIV to the list, so that the Helms amendment would simply "provide an incentive" to modify the list promptly. He added that "other countries have already begun testing for AIDS." (He neglected to name the countries: Belgium, Bulgaria, China, Costa Rica, Cuba, Czechoslovakia, India, Iraq, Kuwait, Saudi Arabia, South Africa, South Korea, the Soviet Union, Thailand, and the United Arab Emirates.)

Former Senator Lowell Weicker of Connecticut, a liberal, and frequent Helms foe, raised an objection. If the President has already directed the PHS to add HIV to the list, he wondered, why then was an amendment needed? Perhaps he anticipated a problem: If an act of Congress now added HIV to the list, would another act of Congress be needed to remove it subsequently? But Weicker quickly moved on, dropping his objection to the amendment and concentrating instead on removing the link between the contagious disease list and the AZT appropriations bill. Helms conceded the point, and a voice vote was taken on the motion to add HIV to the list of dangerous contagious diseases by Congressional statute. The result: unanimous—97 yeas, no nays.

A careful perusal of the Senate debate demonstrates the reasons for the landslide vote. First, though the amendment was eventually separated from the AZT funding bill, Helms was exercising his porcupine power, threatening to block passage of an important AIDS bill. Second, whether or not the PHS was politically coerced into doing so (many have claimed that it was), the agency was on record as wanting to add HIV to the list. Before voting yes, Senator Weicker, a longtime AIDS advocate, said: "I will vote for the amendment . . . not because it is the amendment of the distinguished Senator from North Carolina, but because it is a recommendation of the Public Health Service."

Finally, and most important, the floor debate reveals that the Senators (probably even Senator Helms) thought they were talking about limiting the ability of HIV-infected people to *immigrate*, not to *travel*, to the United States. Said Helms:

"The Federal Government has the obligation to protect its citizenry from foreigners emigrating to this country who carry deadly diseases which threaten the health and safety of U.S. citizens." Added Senator Danforth of Missouri: "Clearly, the United States does now reserve the right to exclude from our borders people who would emigrate here, on the basis that they carry communicable diseases. Clearly, AIDS is a communicable disease. . . ."

And so, on June 2, 1987, HIV became the eighth "dangerous and contagious disease" on the list carried by all U.S. immigration officials. One such official was checking incoming passengers through customs at Minneapolis–St. Paul International Airport on April 2, 1989. And one such passenger was Hans Paul Verhoef.

At the time of Verhoef's detention by the INS, about ten HIV-infected visitors had previously been denied entry into the U.S. under the provisions of the Helms amendment. These individuals, not wishing to do battle with the U.S. government, simply reboarded their planes and returned to their native countries. But Verhoef was different. "You can't stop a virus at the border," he said in justifying his legal challenge, "any more than you can catch water with a net."

Verhoef was taken to Scott County jail, where he was forced to don prison stripes and shackles. Two days later, after extensive media attention that embarrassed jail officials, Verhoef was moved to the hospital ward of Oak Park Correction Facility, a maximum-security prison. A gay rights legal group filed a waiver to allow him admission into the United States. And then he waited.

When the INS wrote its regulations clarifying the Helms amendment in 1987, it left open the possibility of waivers. For individuals excluded by the INS (for whatever reason), the agency traditionally grants waivers for family unity, for humanitarian reasons, or because doing so would be in the public interest. Moreover, said the INS, HIV-infected individuals applying for a waiver needed to satisfy three additional conditions:

1. The danger to the public health of the United States created by the alien's admission is minimal.
2. The possibility of the spread of the infection created by the alien's admission is minimal.
3. There will be no cost incurred by any government agency as a result of the alien's admission.

An immigration newsletter characterized these criteria as "an extremely strict test for qualifying for a waiver" and predicted that few aliens would meet all three conditions.

Undaunted, Verhoef and his attorneys pressed on. On April 6, 1989, four days after Verhoef was imprisoned, the INS district director in Bloomington, Minnesota, recommended approval of the waiver. The official wrote that Verhoef was "a mature individual who is significantly involved in the prevention of AIDS. [He] has indicated that he will not engage in any unsafe behavior in the United States. . . ." But the Washington office of the INS refused to sign the waiver. In overruling his district director, Associate INS Commissioner Richard Norton wrote that "the risk of harm by an AIDS-infected alien, in the absence of humanitarian reasons for permitting the temporary admission of aliens, far outweighs the privilege of an alien to enter the United States to participate in a conference."

Verhoef later told the *Village Voice* that officials seemed particularly interested in the sex toys that the Netherlander claimed to use in safe-sex education. The INS attorney, Verhoef recalled, "would pick up the toys and ask, 'Is this a hundred percent safe? Yes or no?' He wanted me to promise that I wouldn't have sex when I was in the U.S., and I refused to do that. I know very well how AIDS is transmitted and how it's not. I told him, 'People with AIDS need caressing and hugging too. When does [that] stop and sex start? Perhaps you can tell me.' His ears got very red.''

Later that day, administrative law judge Robert Vinikoor overruled the INS and approved Verhoef's waiver, allowing him to enter the United States. The INS, engaged in what Lyndon Johnson liked to call a pissing contest, issued an emergency appeal of the ruling. After this was promptly denied by the Board of Immigration Appeals, Verhoef boarded a plane and arrived in San Francisco at 9:32 P.M. A hero's welcome awaited him.

That none of the conference organizers, myself included, really noticed the Verhoef drama as it was being played out in Minnesota was testimony to our myopia and naiveté at the time. We were hard at work putting together our *Call for Abstracts and Registration*, a document describing major conference policies and the procedure for submitting new scientific research for review. For the document to be ready for distribution in Montreal in June 1989 required that it be at the printer by mid-April. We were also in the midst of interviewing candidates for both media and community-relations director, either of whom might have warned us of the coming storm.

But our workload was not as determining a factor as our naiveté. We saw ourselves as scientists planning a scientific conference; the Verhoef case was a *political* issue. We quickly passed over the stories about Verhoef in the newspaper in deference to others on AIDS vaccine research and epidemic trends in Brazil.

When we did take notice of it, we saw the Verhoef case as an embarrassment to the U.S. and an example of the laws that result when politicians fail to listen to scientific and medical facts: HIV is simply not casually contagious, and can only be contracted by identifiable high-risk activity. Somehow, shockingly, we failed to see the connection between the Verhoef case and the Sixth International Conference on AIDS.

That is, not until two days after Verhoef's arrival in San Francisco—the day Randy Shilts's weekly column appeared in the *San Francisco Chronicle*. Shilts painted a horrifying scenario: that hundreds of HIV-infected people might be arrested on their way to *our* conference. Prisons in the Bay Area would not be large enough to contain them all, necessitating the construction of makeshift internment camps to detain conference registrants. "This scenario gave conference organizers nightmares all last week," Shilts wrote. "Already the consensus has emerged among AIDS experts and international health officials: If the immigration policy remains in place, the San Francisco conference should be cancelled and moved elsewhere."

Shilts's style of advocacy journalism was at work. At the time his column was published, we did not know of a single "AIDS expert" or "international health official" who favored cancelling or relocating the conference. But the concept, once sanctified by the nation's top AIDS writer, took on a life of its own. We had not had nightmares in the previous week, but we would develop them in the weeks to come.

Even fourteen months before D-day, moving the conference was an impossibility. Finding a convention center able to accommodate ten to fifteen thousand people must be done at least two years in advance. Reserving more than ten thousand hotels rooms in one city—this too could not be done on short notice. Finally, and perhaps most important, a meeting of the magnitude of the International AIDS Conference requires a sponsor with deep pockets. It had taken substantial effort for Ziegler and Volberding to convince the UCSF administration to bankroll the conference, since the administrators knew they would spend nearly two million dollars before seeing their first dollar of revenue. Clearly, the university would not be willing to risk millions of dollars for a conference in Amsterdam or Geneva. Just as clearly, there would be no way to come up with an alternate sponsor in the next few months.

* * *

A week or so after Verhoef's arrival, a member of a local working group on immigration asked me to speak to the group about the conference's position on the Helms amendment. I wandered into the meeting innocently expecting a sympathetic audience. After all, we had nothing to do with the law; we were just doctors and researchers trying to plan a conference. The people in the working group were the lawyers and politicians.

It didn't take long for me to recognize that our perception of the situation bore no resemblance to that of the AIDS activists, politicians, and lawyers in the room. For a long while I sat quietly as the conference organizers took it from both barrels. The speakers' points were:

1. Passively opposing the law, as we had done, was inadequate. We needed to be in there slugging it out with the U.S. government. "Don't underestimate the power you have as respected scientists and clinicians to influence policy," one said.

2. A waiver of the regulation for conference delegates would be insufficient. Only a repeal of the entire law, so that all HIV-infected travelers could enter freely, would do.

3. Even though they could see the benefits of having the conference in San Francisco, they were willing to see it moved (or even cancelled) over the travel issue.

4. If the conference wasn't moved and the regulations remained in place, we could expect ugly, potentially violent demonstrations. I was reminded that, by a fluke of scheduling, our conference would take place during Gay and Lesbian Freedom Week, which traditionally draws hundreds of thousands of gays to the streets of San Francisco. "What do you say to an eight-hundred-pound gorilla?" rhetorically asked Jim Foster, veteran

gay activist and member of San Francisco's Health Commission. "You say, 'Yes sir.' We're that eight-hundred-pound gorilla."

The group's anger and frustration were palpable. My trip into the lion's den had not been eased by John Ziegler's interview in the *San Francisco Examiner* the previous week. John's background was not that of an activist. He hailed from a Republican family, sported an Amherst diploma, and had logged more than two decades in the employ of the U.S. government, first at the National Cancer Institute and now at the San Francisco Veteran's Hospital. He had been involved in AIDS from the beginning, and was one of the first to recognize the association between AIDS and tumors of the lymph system. He is a caring and compassionate physician. But none of this had prepared him for the politics of AIDS in San Francisco's gay community. It was not that I had any less to learn than did John; it was that he, being twenty years my senior, had much more to unlearn.

Ziegler told the *Examiner* that, while he sympathized with activists who wished to change the immigration law, the San Francisco meeting would be "a world *scientific* conference intended to exchange research and information and show the progress being made toward cure and prevention. The conference is not intended for persons with AIDS or HIV infection," he added. The *Examiner* interview was the equivalent of starving the lions in the den and then kicking them in the butt.

Jim Foster, who had AIDS himself, was livid over Ziegler's interview. He lectured me for thirty minutes about the necessity of moving the conference out of the country if the law was not changed. Finally, having begun to regain my poise after my unanticipated hazing, I spoke up. My voice trembling slightly, I told Foster that moving the conference was logistically impossible, and those who favored this course needed to admit that they were actually talking about cancelling it. Second, cancelling the conference would come at a great cost, as it serves as the major forum for the discussion of new scientific information related to AIDS and HIV infection. And third, we agreed that the policy was unsupported by scientific evidence and just plain wrong. Finally, I told the group that we were more than willing to work with the community in any way possible to try to change the immigration law.

It was in that room, seething with tension and mistrust, that the fragile coalition was born. I think everyone present recognized the potential power of a union between the scientists and the activists, but also recognized that the path to such a union was studded with obstacles. As I left the room, Pat Christen, Executive Director of the San Francisco AIDS Foundation, thanked me for my input and acknowledged my courage in subjecting myself to the excoriation. She was too charitable. Had I known what I was in for, I probably would not have attended. In any case, I left the room a lot more politically savvy than I had been when I walked in.

I met with Ziegler and Volberding the next day. We knew that a change in strategy was necessary if the conference was to survive. No more statements about the meeting being primarily "scientific"—both because such statements represented political suicide and because they set up a false dichotomy. Larry Bush, San Francisco Mayor Art Agnos's gay community advisor and speechwriter, put it starkly: "A number of the major researchers of world stature are themselves infected with AIDS. There is no line that says on one side are patients and on another sit physicians. . . . People with AIDS are not human petri dishes to be treated as an asset in a researcher's application for grants."

It was also clear to us that the conference needed to become much more aggressive in fighting the law and in engaging concerned scientists in a "high road" assault on the public health flaws of the immigration regulations. We began writing letters to major political figures detailing our strong objection to the law on public health grounds, and informing them of the real possibility of the conference's cancellation. We also planned a series of meetings with local AIDS representatives to try to forge a cooperative, instead of an adversarial, relationship.

Over the next two to three weeks, our strategy began to bear fruit. Commentary in the gay papers in San Francisco began to focus on Washington instead of the conference as the major culprit. Our subsequent meetings with AIDS community groups became much more productive as we recognized our unity of interest. The groups, we were gratified to learn, had a strong interest in keeping the conference in San Francisco and were willing to work with us to ensure this outcome. Our message that the conference could not be moved began to sink in.

The use of the conference as a lever to effect political change, although initially unpleasant for us, was understandable. But what if push came to shove? What if the conference did get cancelled over a political issue? And what if HIV-infected people who might have received lifesaving treatment information were not given that opportunity because the single best forum for the dissemination of scientific information was obliterated? This was the other message that we began to deliver to the local groups. Sure, the bathwater stinks, but the baby could really be something special. In an article entitled, "Will the AIDS Conference Be Cancelled?" in the *Chronicle*, I said, "The conference can save lives. Cancelling it won't." Randy Shilts agreed. "At this point, only one thing seems sure," Shilts wrote. "Moving the conference from San Francisco means cancelling the gathering altogether. . . . Just who wins in that scenario is unclear."

The most challenging convert was Jim Foster. Foster persisted with his plan to bring a resolution before the San Francisco Department of Public Health to withdraw the Department's cosponsorship of the meeting. At the time, the Department had neither given nor promised us any money, so we were not terribly concerned about the fiscal impact of its withdrawal. But we were gravely concerned about the message it might send. A perception that the conference might soon be cancelled could easily snowball into a self-fulfilling prophecy, as prospective staff, scientists, and donors abandoned a sinking ship.

We met with Foster and outlined a potential scenario if the Department of Public Health withdrew. We claimed, only with slight overstatement, that UCSF was sure to follow suit given its wary sponsorship of the meeting and aversion to fiscal risks. If this were to occur, the conference would be cancelled. Foster, an astute politician, quickly realized that he would be perceived as personally responsible for the cancellation of the 1990 conference. He paused for a moment, then graciously offered to delay his Health Commission resolution for a week. "But keep this totally confidential; I don't want the media to know I've backed off," Foster said. We said good-bye at the door, and awaited our next appointment, with local television reporter Jim Bunn. "I saw Jim Foster on his way out," Bunn remarked when he arrived. "He says he's holding off on the Health Commission resolution." So much for confidentiality.

Although the tide was turning in our favor locally, we were still battling the clock and desperately needed some action in Washington. Montreal was a mere three weeks away, and rumors were flying that the international gay community would challenge the INS regulations both in Montreal and at the annual Gay and Lesbian Freedom Day Parade in San Francisco. According to these rumors, five hundred people with AIDS would proudly proclaim their HIV status to immigration officials as they crossed the United States border. If these people were all arrested, the 1990 conference would be cancelled. Even if we tried to continue planning, our ability to raise funds would be decimated, and both the World Health Organization and the International AIDS Society would withdraw their sponsorship. Furthermore, none of us were particularly interested in planning a meeting whose two most memorable aspects were hundreds of thousands of screaming protestors and scores of registrants languishing in maximum security prisons.

It was against this backdrop that we hired Dana Van Gorder. Dana had first come to us months earlier to interview for the position of Director of Communications. He was impressive—a compact, enthusiastic, and savvy man in his early thirties who understood the politics of AIDS and the gay community as well as anyone. He was openly gay himself; this was vital for our relationship with the local community.

Dana's main experience was in the political sphere. He had been an aide to San Francisco Supervisor Harry Britt in the early 1980s, becoming enmeshed in the fierce debates over closing the gay bathhouses. Later, he organized the campaign against Proposition 102 in California. That proposition, sponsored by right-wing Congressman William Dannemeyer, would have mandated tracing the contacts of every HIV-positive individual in the state. Dana mobilized one of the first coalitions of concerned scientists and AIDS advocates to fight the law on public health grounds, and successfully defeated the proposition. At Dana's interview for Communications Director, we were struck by his talent and heart, but felt that he lacked the experience to organize a press operation for two thousand journalists. At the time of this first interview, we were also hard put to see the direct relevance of his political experience to our needs. After all, we were planning a scientific conference.

How times had changed. Now we realized that his expertise—the ability to mobilize scientists and the community in an effective public relations campaign against an ill-conceived law—was precisely what we needed. Dana was hired to direct community relations for the conference, ostensibly to deal with the immigration issue. We now had a field general. Our sleepy political machine was finally ready to spring into action.

An endless string of letters, memos, and press releases authored by Dana flew across my desk for approval. He gave Ziegler, Volberding, and me long lists of scientists to telephone for support in battling the immigration policy. The calls began early in the morning and went on late into the night, from our offices and homes. The phone ambush continued even into my barber's chair, where my beeper sounded for the thousandth time. "Dr. Jonathan Mann," my barber announced, "returning your call." Jonathan (whose travel schedule would make a Presidential candidate cower) was in the waiting lounge at de Gaulle Airport in Paris, on his way to Uganda where he would not have access to a phone for several days. Yelling over the noise of wailing blow-dryers, Mann informed us that our efforts were beginning to pay off. A few days earlier, he had met with Louis Sullivan, U.S. Secretary of Health and Human Services, and James Mason, Assistant Secretary of Health and Director of the Public Health Service. The HIV-travel issue was now being debated at the highest levels of the Justice, Health and Human Services, and Immigration Departments, as well as at the White House. Mann felt confident that a reinterpretation of the immigration ruling was forthcoming, one in which HIV-infected people would be allowed to enter the United States to attend scientific conferences. This was not as far as he wanted the U.S. to go, but it would at least allow his agency, the World Health Organization, to continue its cosponsorship of San Francisco.

We received a similarly hopeful message the next day at a meeting with San Francisco Congresswoman Nancy Pelosi. Speaking to conference organizers, representatives of the U.S. Public Health Service, and San Francisco city administrators, Pelosi discouraged the group from trying to return to the Senate to repeal the Helms amendment. A trip to the Senate to change the law, she said, might get the wrong people (read: Helms and other conservatives) interested in the issue. "We could end up with something worse than we have now," she added. Everyone at the meeting agreed to continue pushing for a reinterpretation of the regulations by INS or the Public Health Service—to get the agencies to agree that HIV infection was not casually contagious and therefore the regulations should not apply to travelers. The representative of the Health Service indicated that such a change was in the offing.

On May 18, 1989, six weeks after Hans Paul Verhoef had innocently arrived at Minneapolis International Airport, the Justice Department announced a policy change. As before, the INS (a branch of the Justice Department) would use a "balancing test" to determine whether the benefits of admitting an HIV-infected alien outweighed the risk to the public health and possible drain on U.S. tax dollars. If so, the INS would grant a waiver of the "dangerous and contagious" restriction, and would stamp the alien's passport with a number—212 (d)(3)(a)(6)—that indicated a waiver had been granted.

The change, announced INS Commissioner Alan Nelson, was that criteria for demonstrating "a sufficient public benefit" would be relaxed. HIV-infected aliens would now be permitted to travel to the United States to attend conferences, obtain medical treatment, conduct business, or visit relatives. However, travel for the purpose of tourism was deemed not to "constitute the requisite public benefit to overcome the risk."

The reaction to the Justice Department announcement, and the May 25 INS cable clarifying the new regulations, was lukewarm. We quickly wrote Attorney General Richard Thornburgh and Health Secretary Louis Sullivan urging them to go further—to lift all restrictions on travel by HIV-infected people. The International AIDS Society prepared a statement for Montreal that would commit the organization to planning no future conferences in countries restricting travel of people with AIDS, thus endangering the 1992 conference scheduled for Boston.

Despite the calls for further change, the new regulations took the wind out of the sails of those lobbying on the travel issue. The original objections were voiced because HIV-infected people would be unable to attend the Sixth International Conference; the recent changes meant that they could attend. The paperwork for a waiver was inconvenient, certainly, and the thirty- to sixty-day waiting period a nuisance. But the primary objection to the law had been answered.

Although we were disappointed that the government had not done more, we were relieved that the changes would allow our conference planning to go forward. We heard little talk about cancelling our meeting during the Montreal conference. Our two months as political lobbyists had been exhilarating and productive. But we were now ready to return to the real task at hand. Enough politics.

When the INS spoke of applying a "balancing test" in implementing the new policy, it referred to the risks and benefits of an individual HIV-infected traveler entering the U.S. Yet, in formulating the changes, the Bush administration applied another balancing test, one as old as politics itself. The Administration responded to the concerns of AIDS scientists and activists with what they hoped would be enough change to satisfy them and prevent the humiliating cancellation of the San Francisco conference—all without inciting a storm of protest from conservatives. Like tightrope walkers, the White House, Justice, and Health Department policymakers sought refuge in equilibrium. The summer and fall of 1989 passed with neither AIDS groups nor conservatives voicing strenuous objections to the new policy. Administration officials congratulated themselves on passing their balancing test. No one realized that the test was also being graded in Europe, and the results—failure—would take some months to be announced.

5 EMPOWERMENT

Our brief experience as political lobbyists taught us the necessity of working with the local community as we continued our planning. After my initial pummeling by the working group on immigration, we began meeting regularly with three community leaders: Pat Christen of the San Francisco AIDS Foundation, Paul Boneberg of Mobilization Against AIDS, and Ben Schatz of the National Gay Rights Advocates. Two other gay people with AIDS (PWAs), Pierre Ludington, the Executive Director of the American Association of Physicians for Human Rights, and Leon McKusick, a prominent San Francisco psychologist and researcher at UCSF's Center for AIDS Prevention Studies, were invited to serve on our Local Organizing Committee. Over time, the shroud of mistrust between the conference organizers (representing "the scientists") and these individuals (representing "the community") began to lift.

After the divisiveness of Montreal, we wished to expand this informal group into a "community advisory committee" for the conference. It struck me that there were some critical issues such a committee would want to tackle: developing policies regarding admission to the conference for PWAs, providing AIDS information to those unable to attend the meeting, recommending speakers and topics for conference sessions, and liaising with the Gay and Lesbian Freedom Day Parade Committee. We selected Leon McKusick and Pierre Ludington to chair this committee, and chose Dana to be its executive secretary. We left it to these three to come up with a suitable membership.

The committee, as finally constituted, was a rainbow coalition. A number of prominent gay activists from around the city were on it, including members of ACT UP. There were Latinos, blacks, Asians, and American Indians. Lesbians were represented, as were prostitutes. There were even one or two heterosexual men—making the committee a true example of "political correctness."

I looked forward to its first meeting with some anticipation, since there was so much work to be done and the committee seemed uniquely suited to provide us with input. But input was not our only motive in forming the committee. We also needed its members to be on our side if push came to shove with the activists. Scientists telling ACT UP New York to "play nice" would be an exercise in futility. However, if a community group with strong activist ties was sufficiently invested in the conference, it could serve as a vital buffer against ACT UP's brand of guerrilla street theater.

On July 25, 1989, some thirty community representatives filed into the conference room at the San Francisco AIDS Foundation for the first meeting of the "Community Advisory Committee" of the Sixth International Conference on AIDS. The meeting was a fiasco. Three hours of process, procedure, and politics. "They've brought us together to fuck with us!" "The conference is being run by lily-white men." "We need access to the Executive Committee." "We must be empowered!"

The word "empowered" is a buzzword, almost a cliché, in the AIDS activist community—the community's reaction to many years of repression. An empowered PWA seizes control of his own destiny and becomes an active participant in his own care. The concept is commendable, but also problematic. For in the hands of its most ardent proponents, it completely denies the possibility of another's expertise. The empowered PWA or activist need not heed the counsel of physician, nurse, or researcher. To question such advice is doubtless healthy, but to reject it out of hand as a threat to empowerment, as some do, seems foolhardy.

This group was big on empowerment. Hank Wilson, from People with AIDS San Francisco, pushed the community group to choose one chairperson who would also serve on the conference's major committees. "With this," he said, "we will be able to kill—make that empower—two birds with one stone."

The committee was not about to take substantive action on any issues before being suitably empowered. They demanded representation on every conference committee, including all four of the scientific program committees. After the Fifth International Conference, we had spent weeks reassuring basic scientists that ours would be a productive, scientific meeting free from the distractions of Montreal. Now we were entertaining demands from AIDS activists to sit and vote on committees judging research in basic immunology and molecular genetics. How can we possibly make this thing work, I wondered.

What worried me most was that their wants appeared insatiable. On every issue they demanded more access, more community involvement, more empowerment. Our work with them on the immigration issue seemed to count for nothing. The scientific community's protestations over the political atmosphere of Montreal would not temper their demands. Nor would the international nature of the meeting induce them to look beyond their parochial concerns.

I prodded them for some tangible recommendations. "Change the committee's name to the 'Community Task

Force,' " they said. "We are not advisory." They demanded that we waive the $400 conference admission fee for hundreds of PWAs. Finally, they wanted a mandate. We had requested their input on about a dozen major issues, but this did not constitute the requisite mandate. Only if something was called a mandate, apparently, was it a mandate.

The next day, Dana, Leon, Pierre and I brought the community group's recommendations back to the conference's Local Organizing Committee for comment. A few on the Organizing Committee, including Cochair Paul Volberding, objected to dropping the "advisory" from the group's title. "We will try to gather their input and use it in a way that's productive," said Volberding. "But we need to be blunt. This *is* an advisory group. They can't have representation on every committee. We will understand if they find our conditions unacceptable and choose to go elsewhere. But we will not give in on every point."

Most of the "mandates" suggested by the community group were acceptable to the Organizing Committee. "Mandate F," in particular, was a syntactical *tour de force*: "To recommend ways to provide opportunities for AIDS activist organizations to present their public policy and political agenda at the time of the conference." We were encouraged, because the recommendation committed us only to providing visibility for the activists "at the time of the conference" and not within the conference walls.

Despite some initial balking by the Organizing Committee, virtually all of the mandates were promptly accepted until the ninth. The community group insisted that it be allowed to review and possibly publish the abstracts (research summaries submitted to the conference for review) rejected by the conference's scientific committees. The scientists felt strongly that the quality of the science presented at the meeting needed to be upgraded; to do this required more selectivity in judging abstracts. Whereas Montreal rejected fewer than 10 percent of the 5,900 abstracts they received, our committee wanted a rejection rate of 40 or 50 percent. Scientists on our committee also voiced concerns about resurrecting rejected abstracts, since many researchers might want to submit them to other meetings, and they couldn't do this if they had already been published by the Task Force.

The community's perspective was completely different, focussing narrowly on the case of Compound Q. A derivative of a Chinese cucumber root, "Q" showed anti-HIV activity in test tubes; the community impatiently awaited more results. However, a sketchy abstract on the compound was one of the few papers rejected by the Montreal conference. To many of the activists this example represented the danger inherent in too much selectivity—"lifesaving research" might be overlooked either through oversight or malice on the part of the Program Committee. The Local Organizing Committee left me with the unenviable task of developing a solution to this problem. I stalled, but eventually allowed a Task Force member to review the rejected abstracts and contact authors for permission to reprint them in a nonconference publication.

The community group's two final recommendations were its most contentious. In order to have access to the decision-making apparatus of the conference, they demanded representation on each of our program committees. Although this would not be a problem on the Track C epidemiology and Track D policy committees (in fact, a few members of the Task Force already attended those committees' meetings), we worried about placing an activist on the basic science committee. The Organizing Committee counterproposed that the community group submit a list of qualified individuals to sit on each of the scientific committees. For the basic science committee, this meant that the community group needed to find an individual qualified to review abstracts in basic immunology and virology. Of course, the Task Force promptly submitted a suitable candidate.

Weeks earlier, after recognizing that the Local Organizing

Committee, with its twenty-five diverse members and monthly meetings, was incapable of making day-to-day decisions, we developed the concept of a compact "executive committee." This group, with five to seven members, would meet frequently and render decisions related to budget and administration. When the Task Force saw "Executive Committee" atop a revised conference organizational chart, they demanded membership. In this highly politicized environment, the Executive Committee would not stand up to the light of day. It lacked the breadth of the Local Organizing Committee. More important, it was too small to handle the presence of one or two vocal activists and still conduct business. Recognizing these problems, the Local Organizing Committee promptly voted the newly formed Executive Committee out of business before its first meeting. The community group did not need representation on a committee that was now defunct.

Despite negotiating and finessing away a few of these demands, the Organizing Committee had acceded to most of the community's recommendations. In so doing, it had rejected the sentiments of some of its most prominent scientists. Would there be an end to the protests? Or would there be an ever-increasing list of demands, today's concession being forgotten by tomorrow? The answer would determine the course of our conference, the feasibility of future conferences, and the tone of the relationship between the scientist and activist communities in years to come.

The second meeting of the Community Task Force two weeks later was more of the same. It wasn't just that Task Force members mistrusted the scientists and the conference organizers; they mistrusted each other too. Some members became incensed after learning that others had met "behind their backs." One gay Asian male complained that the other gay Asian male in the group did not adequately represent his interests nor those of the gay Asian male community. A black woman in the group, noting that the only PWAs on the Local Organizing Committee were gay white men, complained that there were "no people of color and no ovaries" in the conference organization. Task Force members insisted on selecting their own chairs, but were unable to decide on who they should be.

Even the food was a source of controversy. As with the first meeting, Dana brought an appetizing and, we thought, politically correct selection of mineral waters and vegetables. One of the few supportive members of the group took me aside. "You really shouldn't be too extravagant with the food," she whispered. "They won't believe you when you tell them you don't have money for their favorite projects."

Finally, after suffering through two more hours of process issues, I spoke up. "The conference will take place on June 20 to 24, 1990. Our timeline is unforgiving." I then went on to describe the major decisions facing us, including choices for keynote speakers and attempts at community outreach. "My hope is that you folks will finish the procedural issues and move on to making hard choices by the time decisions come due. However, if not, I promise you that we'll make the decisions without your input." The Task Force responded with a few minutes of focussed work, before lapsing into the default mode of process deliberations.

Once again, I finished the meeting drained and exhausted, and was in an irascible mood the next day. Our commitment to involving the community in the conference was genuine, but the Task Force was going nowhere. Leon McKusick, Pierre Ludington, and Dana Van Gorder were equally frustrated.

The four of us met for breakfast a few days later at a lovely flower-filled cafe in the heart of the Castro District, the center of gay life in San Francisco. My education continued—I had little doubt that I was the only heterosexual person in the restaurant. I watched with amusement as my three companions' eyes followed in tandem when a handsome man entered the restaurant. When another man ordered breakfast seemingly oblivious of the parakeet sitting on his shoulder, I knew I was not in Kansas anymore.

The three gay men were finding themselves in an increasingly awkward position. While they were highly critical of the atmosphere at the Task Force meetings (Pierre called many of the participants "process divas"), they were equally angry at the Local Organizing Committee, which often derided the community group as too political and scientifically unsophisticated. None of us voiced the concern we all shared: that the three moderate gay men would, over time, find themselves stranded on an island in the middle of the widening river separating the two camps—too scientific and allied with the researchers to be credible representatives of the community, and too much a product of the community to be fully embraced by the scientists. The cries of "Uncle Tom," I thought sadly, might not be far away.

In his 1961 book *Political Influence*, political scientist Edward Banfield described two paradigms for decision-making in complex political environments. In the "central decision" paradigm, choices are made by a central authority (e.g., chairman, mayor, or executive board) who tries to realize some goal for the group. The advantages of this paradigm—that it provides for efficiency and, at least potentially, the "best outcome for all"—are often outweighed by its fundamental flaw: People don't take kindly to being ruled.

An alternative, the "social choice" paradigm, produces decisions as the accidental by-product of a tug-of-war (usually verbal and psychological) between two or more interested parties, who often share no common goal and who make their choices competitively and without regard to each other. Every mayor or committee chair learns the importance of considering (or at least giving lip service to) social choice before rendering decisions. The flaw in the social choice paradigm is that the most ardent proponents of a position, who typically shout the loudest, often thwart the goals of the majority. "It is the necessity of constantly making such concessions," Banfield observed, "of giving everyone something so as to generate enough support to allow any action at all, that makes government policy so lacking in comprehensiveness and consistency."

Banfield recognized a middle ground, the "mixed decision-choice" process. In this paradigm, the interested parties are allowed to duke it out, each seeking competitive advantage. But there is also a central decision-maker who intervenes in the selection process by coordinating the activities of the parties and limiting their framework for discussion. Though stressful for the decision-maker, who lacks the central decision model's autonomy and the freedom to simply ratify the results of the social choice brawl, the mixed decision-choice model is optimal given a democratic system, Banfield and others have judged. And as Churchill said of democracy, it is the worst system . . . except for all the others.

As the interested parties—the Community Task Force and the Local Organizing Committee—struggled for advantage, I found myself in the position of central decision-maker, trying to constrain the groups' choices and facilitate the decision process. Banfield gave me hope: "That the mixed-decision-choice process . . . takes more time to produce an outcome than, presumably, a central decision process would take and that the outcome, when reached, is likely to be a stalemate cannot, of course, be held against it. Time spent discovering and evaluating the probable consequences of a proposal is not necessarily wasted; and if in the end nothing is done, or not much is done, that may be because it is in the public interest to do little or nothing."

Clearly, nothing was being done by the Task Force. But I remained unconvinced that this was in the public—or its own—interest.

* * *

When I came home after the third meeting of the Community Task Force, my wife noticed that I was not swearing. "Was the meeting cancelled?" she wondered.

Magically, the Task Force had finally listened to my admonitions and recognized that there was work to be done, work that could not await another six hours of dickering. The presence of Paul Boneberg, director of Mobilization Against AIDS, was vital. Boneberg is an extremely committed activist, but also a voice of reason. The meeting began with a vote for a cochair to serve alongside Shirley Gross, the minority advocate selected as one of the chairs at the second meeting. I braced myself for another harangue against Pierre Ludington and Leon McKusick for being "flunkies" of the conference since both had UCSF affiliations and already served on the Local Organizing Committee. But Boneberg preempted the objections. "If we select either Pierre or Leon, we'll send a strong message to the conference organizers that the Task Force wants to cooperate," he said. Members nodded their heads in agreement and promptly selected McKusick as cochair. The Task Force then selected representatives to each of the scientific committees; this process too was remarkably painless. Each of the committee's representatives were reasonable people who added a new perspective and important ethnic and gender diversity. Mike Shriver, an HIV-infected member of ACT UP, spoke about community access to the conference, and recommended that we help organize roundtable discussions involving prominent members of the scientific and PWA community at a community site. His subcommittee had researched the idea and even conducted site visits to potential venues. The rest of the Task Force, clearly impressed by the good work of Shriver's subcommittee, congratulated him and approved the recommendation.

The Community Task Force had finally proven itself to be capable of substantive work. The report by Shriver's small subcommittee on community access transformed the attitude of the rest of the members, many of whom, like me, had grown weary of the politicking and processing. At once, the mood elevated, people began to volunteer for positions, and Task Force meetings became genial and energized. We would eventually clash again, most memorably over the Task Force's demand that we distribute twelve hundred free Conference passes (one-tenth of our anticipated registration) to PWAs. But during these later clashes, the Task Force would question the degree of our commitment to PWA and activist inclusion, not the essence of that commitment itself. The third meeting proved to be a turning point for the Task Force—and for the conference.

Upon leaving the meeting, a few ACT UP members collegially told me of their plans to target one of the large drug companies for "price-gouging." Jokingly, I asked them to hold off until the company had paid for its exhibit booth space. "We'll try," said one, laughing. "When do you expect the money?" I left the meeting cheered by this new sense of cooperation and feeling that I might grow to understand their perspective. I was convinced that such understanding was critical to our chances of planning a successful conference.

6 THE GAUNTLET IS THROWN

Political advocacy and health care are age-old bedfellows. In the 1880s, Clara Barton, founder of the American Red Cross, spent much of her time and energy wooing politicians for support. As political economist James Bennett observed in his 1990 monograph *Health Research Charities: Image and Reality*, major twentieth-century health charities like the American Lung Association and the American Cancer Society, concerned with the preservation of their nonprofit status, downplay their lobbying activities while publicizing their charity work. However, their actions—whether advocating for antismoking legislation or increased NIH funding—speak volumes about their true missions. As one perceptive physician said during the 1913 annual meeting of the National Association for the Study and Prevention of Tuberculosis (forerunner of the American Lung Association), "It is getting difficult relatively to get as much private money as you need, whereas if you strike for public money you can get it in greater and greater abundance. Therefore, we must turn our energies from begging money to voting money."

ACT UP, then, is simply another in a long history of health-related political lobbies. Only the disease is new, not the concept.

On the face of it, this is correct. And yet there is something so singular, so revolutionary about ACT UP that the world of health policy will never be the same. The anger, the youth, the chutzpah, the danger. Perhaps it is the danger—the sense that events stand just a hair's breadth away from chaos— that best captures the attention of the activist's target. It was the danger that gripped us by the neck and shook us from side to side as the conference approached.

The seeds of ACT UP were planted in 1969 at the Stonewall Inn, a Greenwich Village gay bar. It was there that a police raid led to three days of rioting, an event that ushered in the modern gay liberation movement.

By the time the nation's first AIDS cases were reported in the *Morbidity and Mortality Weekly Report* in 1981, American gays had acquired substantial political clout, especially in the urban centers of the east and west coasts. Such power could not be easily quantified by the usual tallies of gay legislators and bureaucrats. The movement resulted in an infrastructure of journalists, businessmen, lawyers, writers, and doctors who had come out of the closet in the previous decade. Many understood the levers of power, and had the collective skills to manipulate these levers. But first, they had to agree on a political agenda.

In the late 1970s, the agenda, to a large degree, was the promotion of sexual freedom. Tragically, this focus rendered the community a set-up for the rapid, epidemic spread of a new virus. To compound the tragedy, few in the gay community foresaw the impending holocaust in the early 1980s, and most concentrated their attention on preserving their hard-won sexual freedom and fighting discrimination against victims of the disease.

Elisabeth Kübler-Ross, in her classic treatise *On Death and*

Dying, observed that individuals progress through five stages when confronted with their own mortality: denial, anger, bargaining, depression, and acceptance. As gays confronted death after numbing death in the early 1980s, the community's reaction seemed transfixed on denial. Gays who called for sexual restraint were often derisively branded "prudes," "monogamists," or, worst of all, "internalized homophobes" by other gays.

New York writer Larry Kramer had been called these things and more after the publication of his 1978 novel, *Faggots*. In it, Kramer chided his community for its emphasis on sexual freedom. "Why do faggots have to fuck so fucking much?" he had written. After the first cases of "gay cancer" spread like wildfire among New York gays, Kramer promoted the same theme: sexual caution. His warnings went unheeded, and the personal attacks on him continued. "I think the concealed meaning of Kramer's emotionalism is the triumph of guilt: that gay men *deserve* to die for their promiscuity," claimed one writer in the *New York Native*, a New York City gay weekly.

In 1981, Kramer, a self-acknowledged hypochondriac, read early reports about the strange illnesses sweeping through the gay community. Along with a few friends, he began to raise money to fund research into the still-unnamed disease. The private effort was critical, since both the government and media were ignoring the strange malady that was killing hundreds of gay men in New York, Los Angeles, and San Francisco. How different the national response would be, many thought, if those dying were heterosexual.

In early 1982, Kramer's fundraising efforts culminated in a meeting in his Fifth Avenue apartment at which a new organization, the Gay Men's Health Crisis (GMHC), was formed. Paul Popham was selected as the group's president. As described by Shilts in *And the Band Played On*, the rest of the group worried that "Kramer's confrontational style would make him an unsuitable president of the group, even though he had taken a leading role in its organization. His very name was anathema among the crowd they needed to reach if they were to raise substantial funds."

Kramer and the rest of the GMHC organization soon diverged over strategy. Although the causative virus was still two years away from discovery and the precise mode of transmission had not been elucidated, Kramer was convinced that promiscuity was involved in the spread of the illness. He implored the group to warn gay men of the dangers of what would later be called unsafe sex.

But most of Kramer's fury was directed at the political leadership in New York and Washington. He had quickly moved past denial and into anger—anger over what he perceived as government's indifference to the deaths of large numbers of gay men. Nevertheless, his efforts to goad GMHC into political activism were unsuccessful; the New York group opted to focus its energy on fundraising and education of at-risk populations.

Kramer would later say, "I helped found Gay Men's Health Crisis and watched them turn into a sad organization of sissies. I founded ACT UP and watched them change the world."

Common lore has it that ACT UP began in March 1987 with Kramer's speech to a community group in Greenwich Village. In the speech, he told the audience that two-thirds of them might be dead in five years, casualties of not only a virus but also an unresponsive medical system. "If what you're hearing doesn't rouse you to anger, fury, rage, and action, gay men will have no future here on earth," he fumed.

But Kramer had been saying such things for years. In fact, it's arguable that ACT UP really began in 1982 with one member—Larry Kramer. It may be one of the great tragedies of the epidemic that the organization would not gain its second, third, and thousandth members until the late 1980s, seven years too late.

In short, Larry Kramer, in his 1982 efforts to exhort his

community into political activism, was right. At the time, a few well-placed acts of civil disobedience combined with street theater—the displays that ACT UP would later become famous for—might have jump-started the sleepy medical and health policy establishments into action. But the gay community, fearing a surge in homophobia and a loss of sexual freedom, was reluctant to play up AIDS as a gay disease. So the opportunity was lost. The scientific world, the media, and the government were rarely called to task for ignoring this unprecedented health crisis.

By 1987, it was clear that the feared backlash against gays would not materialize. Certainly, there were examples of shameful discrimination and gay-bashing, but as a whole the gay community's responsible handling of the epidemic had won it sympathy and respect in the straight world. Polls showed a nearly 50 percent increase in the number of Americans who thought homosexuality among consenting adults should be legal and a 20 percent increase in the number who said that gays should have equal job opportunities.

But by 1987 the epidemic had claimed the lives of twenty thousand people in the United States, most of them gay men. In addition, the causative virus had been discovered and HIV tests were widely available, providing many in the gay community evidence of their impending mortality. Although preliminary results of drug trials indicated that effective AIDS treatments were on the horizon, their availability would be governed by the actions of a sluggish and unresponsive federal bureaucracy.

It was in this environment that Kramer's seeds of activism finally took root. Gays finally realized that preventing death was at least as compelling a cause as preserving sexual freedom, and began to mobilize into a political force to be reckoned with. Soon after Kramer's 1987 Greenwich Village speech, ACT UP chapters formed in New York and San Francisco. Described by some as heirs to the traditions of Gandhi and Martin Luther King, Jr., with a touch of Jerry Rubin thrown in, the group's actions were always provocative, often obnoxious, and sometimes amusing. In one protest against government policies, ACT UP hung a piñata resembling Senator Jesse Helms, who was often blamed for the timidity of federal AIDS prevention efforts. Bystanders were invited to take swings at the piñata. When the head finally broke off, condoms rolled out.

Larry Kramer described ACT UP for *Time* magazine as "a street-smart bunch of very courageous scrappers. We have protests. . . . We have telephone zaps where we tie up switchboards. We purchased millions of dollars of tickets when Northwest Airlines refused to carry AIDS people as passengers, tickets that weren't paid for, of course. Because we are gay people and have wonderful taste and can put on wonderful shows, our demonstrations are usually very theatrical."

But 1987 was not 1982. The enemies were now less clear, the battle lines more fluid. In 1982, the targets of Kramer's wrath were the politicians who ignored AIDS and failed to fund research. Now, half a decade later, there were tens of thousands dead from AIDS, hundreds of millions of dollars had been spent, and there was still no cure. The shock and denial of the early 1980s had long passed, replaced by anger and frustration. "My friends die more often than my grandmother's friends do," one young PWA told me. "And she's eighty-six years old."

And so in 1989, the scientists—and the conference—became the target.

The events of Montreal convinced us, if we needed any convincing, that we risked being on the business end of the activists' wrath. But this was San Francisco, a city that had become world-renowned for its AIDS care model by emphasizing cooperation between care providers, patients, government, and the private sector. After the spirit of cooperation began to infuse the meetings of the Community Task Force, we felt increasingly optimistic. This would be the "San Francisco Model" of conferences, we thought.

Watching the eleven o'clock news on September 10, 1989, brought us back to our senses. At the opening of the San Francisco Opera, which, the *San Francisco Chronicle* mused, is "rarely marred by anything more serious than spilled chardonnay," about seventy-five protestors crashed through the glittering crowd. "We're here! We're queer! Stop AIDS NOW!" they shouted. The opening-night crowd became angry and jeered at the demonstrators. Like a scene out of *Casablanca*, audience members sang "The Star-Spangled Banner" at the top of their lungs, trying to drown out the shouts of the activists. There was some punching and shoving, and SWAT officers were called in. One HIV-infected man attending the opera criticized the action. "This is no way to gain attention to the problem of AIDS," he said. "Many people in the audience are the greatest supporters of funding for AIDS-related causes. This is an embarrassment for me as a gay man."

The perpetrators were part of a group called Stop AIDS Now Or Else (SANOE), which had also claimed responsibility for blocking rush-hour traffic on the Golden Gate Bridge eight months earlier. "Since we blocked the Golden Gate Bridge, three of our people have died, and still the power structure has not responded," said a spokesperson for the group. "We know who's in [the opera house]. "The mayor, the governor, and heads of corporations are in there. We want them to use their influence to do something about AIDS."

The opera director, Lotfi Mansouri, took the stage and tried to quiet the crowd, saying: "The San Francisco Opera is noted for its exciting openings, and this is no exception." However, the audience was not amused. "These guys should be prosecuted to the full extent of the law," fumed former Mayor Joseph Alioto, a member of the opening-night crowd. A spokesman for the opera called the demonstration "senseless," noting that the opera had held an AIDS benefit three weeks earlier. "No one has lost more victims to AIDS than the arts organizations, including ours, and as a result we are particularly sensitive to the problem."

Just as the successes of the Community Task Force had lulled us into slumber, the action at the opera snapped us back to attention.

If the night at the opera caused some to question the activists' choice of targets, the attack on New York's St. Patrick's Cathedral in early December 1989 made some wonder who was behind the actions. In his *Chronicle* column, Randy Shilts wrote, "If I didn't know better, I'd swear that the AIDS protestors who have been disrupting services and vandalizing Catholic churches . . . were being paid by some diabolical reactionary group dedicated to discrediting the gay community."

The source of Shilts's scorn began when five thousand demonstrators marched outside the Fifth Avenue cathedral, chanting, "Teach safe sex" and "Just say no is not enough." Events quickly escalated as the protestors—an amalgam of AIDS and abortion rights activists—entered the church to interrupt John Cardinal O'Connor's service. One activist snatched a Communion wafer—which Roman Catholics believe to be the body of Christ—from the hands of a churchgoer and threw it to the floor.

Some of ACT UP's most prominent members criticized the action at St. Patrick's, which was soon followed by similar protests at churches in Los Angeles and San Francisco. Peter Staley, a twenty-eight-year-old former bond trader and ACT UP leader, called the protests an "utter failure" and "a selfish, macho thing." By shifting the focus to issues of religious freedom, Staley continued, the church protests took the spotlight away from AIDS.

But an increasingly militant Larry Kramer praised the actions. "The Church is perceived as being behind the times

not only on abortion but also on sex education and gay
rights," Kramer told *Time* magazine. "Even though it's representing something that is thousands of years old, every once
in a while, you've got to give the machine a lube job."

By 1989, some of ACT UP's members, like Staley, Mark
Harrington, Jim Eigo, and Michelle Roland were regularly
invited to participate in high-level policy discussions regarding AIDS drug trials. Many AIDS policymakers were surprised to learn how articulate and well-informed the activists
were. But the corridors of power that had been pried opened
by the threat of protest would close quickly if ACT UP's
actions became too confrontational. So ACT UP denied responsibility for the St. Patrick's protest, just as it had with
the opera. It seemed that the activist group did not want to
be too closely associated with unpopular radical actions.

In fact, 1989 saw an alphabet soup of splinter groups spring
up—and often disappear just as quickly. Groups like SPRAY
(Support Prostitutes Rights Against Yuppies), NASA (Never
Again Silent Army), TANTRUM (Take Action Now to Really
Upset the Masses), PISSED (People with Immune System Diseases), and GRINCH (Gay Retaliation for Inexcusable Neg-
ligence and Criminal Homophobia) were born. Their
members accused the police of infiltrating ACT UP and complained that the larger group's size and bureaucracy limited
aggressive action. Unlike ACT UP's open meetings, SANOE
(the group claiming responsibility for the opera and the bridge
protests) worked in total secrecy. The group recruited by
invitation only, there were no announced meetings, and messages were passed by word of mouth. "We just happen to
show up at the right place at the right time," said one SANOE
member.

AIDS activists had succeeded in creating the ultimate in
deniability. When individual ACT UP members were criticized for going too far, the organization spoke of the group's
anarchy. "We can't control our members," they would say,

shrugging their shoulders. And when an unpopular action was contemplated, a splinter group of ACT UP members would form, coin a clever acronym, and protest. Criticism of the protest would be met with, "This wasn't an ACT UP action." In the same way that ACT UP made groups like GMHC and the San Francisco AIDS Foundation look more temperate, the existence of fringe groups like SANOE made ACT UP members seem like moderate statesmen.

However, this continuous push toward increased radicalism carried a price. Nonactivists working to fight AIDS—volunteers, financial contributors, health care providers, researchers—reacted to actions like the opera and St. Patrick's with frustration and anger. AIDS charities complained of a fall in donations after every controversial protest.

ACT UP properly claimed credit for some positive changes in the fight against AIDS. Their actions at the FDA led to speedier testing and distribution of experimental drugs. Their protests against Burroughs-Wellcome, manufacturer of AZT, led to a 20 percent reduction in the price of the most important anti-AIDS medication. Even some of the recipients of their wrath praised the group's effectiveness. "There's no doubt that they've had an enormous effect," said former New York Health Commissioner Stephen Joseph, who was called a "murderer" in Montreal. "We've basically changed the way we make drugs available in the last year."

The activists' success was, in some ways, predictable. In the history of medicine, there had never before been a politically savvy, unified group that found itself at risk for a deadly disease. Most people with cancer or heart disease find they have little in common except for their illness; they lack a group identity or any prior political agenda. But ACT UP works because gays, already politically mobilized from their gay rights experiences in the 1970s, were organized and prepared to do battle.

As 1989 came to an end, many in the gay community found themselves vigorously debating ACT UP's tactics even while acknowledging the group's impact. Were their more aggressive actions, as Shilts claimed, "politics confused with therapy"? Who were the appropriate targets? Churchgoers? Morning commuters? AIDS researchers? Many noted that the gains in AIDS funding and treatment had not been obtained by protest alone, but also by winning the hearts of many heterosexuals who sympathized with the devastation wrought by AIDS on the gay community. If activists alienated this group, they could lose these friends quickly; louder yelling might then be futile.

As the decade of the 1990s began, AIDS activism neared a dangerous crossroads. As Dana and I entered New York's Lesbian and Gay Community Services Center in Greenwich Village to attend an ACT UP meeting in the fall of 1989, it seemed to us that the roads might very well cross on June 20, 1990, at the opening ceremony of the Sixth International Conference on AIDS.

Dana and I walked nervously into the dingy hall fifteen minutes before the regularly scheduled Monday meeting. Erotic murals, varying in both carnal explicitness and physical decay, covered the walls. A few decrepit ceiling fans turned irregularly, providing the room's only ventilation. More than three hundred people were stuffed into a space meant for two-thirds that number.

The crowd was diverse: While many men wore black leather and earrings, some came in business suits. I guessed that there were about fifty women and almost that many people of color. The average age of the crowd was about thirty, so that Larry Kramer, at age fifty-four, looked the role of elder statesman. "I really want to be a sex symbol," Kramer would later tell me, "but they treat me like a father figure."

A half hour after the scheduled start of the meeting, the main activity at the front of the room was a frustrated attempt to hang the AIDS COALITION TO UNLEASH POWER sign. Finally, the sign hung, the meeting could begin. A man with earrings and flowing shoulder-length hair stood in front. "I know we have a number of new members out there," he said. "I ask you to raise your hands." About thirty to fifty people did, to rousing applause. After telling new members not to vote until they'd attended three meetings, the facilitator continued. "In accordance with the laws of this city, all police officers and government officials are now asked to identify themselves." No one came forward. "Come on, boys, I know you're out there," he chuckled. His assumption that the meeting was infiltrated by nonsympathizers was justifiable, especially since ACT UP had shut down the New York Stock Exchange with a protest during the previous week. It mattered little, an ACT UPer later told me. "All important decisions are made in small subcommittees and not at this forum," he said. "The forum is mostly a sociocultural event—a great place to meet people —and has very little to do with the power structure of the organization."

The facilitator then announced that the "ACT UP boutique" was open for business. It was soon doing a brisk trade selling SILENCE = DEATH T-shirts. On each shirt was the distinctive pink triangle—the symbol of ACT UP—set against a black background. The triangle had one important difference from the one Nazis affixed to homosexuals during World War II; this one pointed up. "We were trying to disavow the victim role," said Avram Finkelstein, who helped design the symbol.

Finally the meeting began in earnest. The recently completed election for New York City mayor topped the sprawling agenda. The week before the meeting, Mayor Edward Koch, who had served twelve years in New York but was unpopular among the AIDS community, lost to David Dinkins, the black borough president from Manhattan. Dinkins was well-liked by the activists. The discussion turned to an upcoming Dinkins rally. "I think we should wait it out and not be too visible at the rally," one person said. "Dinkins might be okay. Let's not get too angry." Another activist stood and was recognized by the facilitator. "I don't trust anybody telling us not to get angry. They're telling us to move to the back of the bus," he said bitterly. "Well, fuck them, I say, fuck them!" If the issue was resolved by the end of the meeting, I certainly didn't notice it.

The atmosphere remained electric. I found myself agreeing with writer David Leavitt, who joined ACT UP after noticing that people only seemed to care when straight people got AIDS. Leavitt wrote in the *New York Sunday Times Magazine*: "What I liked best about ACT UP was its joyousness. It was, according to one of its chants, 'loud and rude and strong and queer.' Here was a room full of people who were refusing to accept the common wisdom that as a population affected by AIDS, they were necessarily doomed and hopeless, their lives defined by death." San Francisco writer Chris Adams echoed similar sentiments. "As late as 1988, the fight against AIDS was largely conducted in a quiet and sober manner," Adams wrote in the *Examiner*. "Patients were heroic role models dealing with hopeless situations." But life in the gay community had become a succession of funerals. "Against this stark background, the radical AIDS activists burst onto the scene. Aroused by the quiet ghosts of the dead, they began to speak out. . . .Their rage may have appeared unfocussed, their targets questionable—but they were making a declaration. As one of the traffic stoppers on the cold, foggy [Golden Gate] bridge later put it, 'Being made comfortable to die is not enough anymore.' "

The ACT UP meeting continued. People stood up in random fashion to make statements about various issues, some of which were connected to AIDS in only the loosest way. A severe-looking woman stood. "A friend of mine died today, and I'm pissed off," she bellowed. She described her friend's death in a nearby intensive care unit, and claimed that the patient was abused by nurses and doctors at the hospital. "I think we should plan an action against this hospital," she said, "I think we should sue their butts off." A brief round of applause and she sat down.

The AIDS conference appeared next on the sprawling agenda. Dana, in his best political tone, stood in front of the crowd and announced that the conference had established a massive community outreach program and an active community task force. This was being done, he continued, to ensure input from people with AIDS, people of color, women and gays and lesbians, and members of other groups affected by the epidemic. He described the program briefly and encouraged anyone with questions or comments to speak to him or me. A brief smattering of applause, and he was done. The agenda moved on. I guessed that, being eight months away, the conference was still too far off, too abstract, to be of great interest to these people, many of whom struggled to live through each day.

But there was one person in the hall who was extremely interested in the conference. While the meeting continued, Dana took me aside to introduce me to Larry Kramer. Kramer had short gray hair, a stubby salt-and-pepper beard, and pursed lips. He sweated profusely, like someone constantly nervous. Kramer came right to the point. "I would really like to give the keynote speech at the end of the opening ceremony." Kramer knew that the opening ceremony would be the conference's most visible event, with extraordinary worldwide press coverage. It was there that the measure of our commitment to PWAs and activists would be taken. Kramer pressed further: "Whose decision is this anyway? Is it your decision?" he asked. I obfuscated, saying that the decision would be made by committee, but that we valued his input. "I'll give a moving speech for everybody, not just the activists," he continued. "It will make them all cry."

* * *

Kramer called me a month later, in November 1989, to continue lobbying for a starring role in the opening ceremony. "Somebody has to get up there and say what is not being done," he said. "I think it should be an ACT UP person from somewhere, because most of the news in the last year has been created by ACT UP."

He knew that we had asked ACT UP/New York's Sixth International Conference committee to submit recommendations for opening ceremony speaker. He also knew that his name, although on the recommended list, came after two other PWAs from ACT UP: Vito Russo and Michael Callen. He described the meeting that had generated the recommendations.

"They were going to choose me. It was a *fait accompli*," he said. "And then the meeting began. As usual, it was chaotic. All of a sudden everybody and his brother was allowed to nominate someone. Names were just flying from everywhere.

"I should be the choice," he continued. "Don't pick somebody safe." Could he recommend anyone else from ACT UP for the job? I asked. He responded quickly: "No." I told him that we'd be considering all of the input in making the decision sometime within two months.

Whenever Kramer's name came up, even in speaking with another person from ACT UP, the reaction was always guarded. "He's a loose cannon," a number of people told me. "You won't have any clue about what he's going to say until he's actually up on the stage." I think Kramer sensed that he was not going to be chosen as the major speaker, and on December 2, 1989, his veneer of civility eroded.

Kramer's December 2 letter was addressed to conference Cochair Paul Volberding. When we received it, we had already finalized our commitment to have at least one ACT UP person address the opening ceremony, but had not decided on who. Although we were leaning toward another New York writer, Vito Russo, we had not completely ruled out inviting Larry Kramer. But we continued to be cautious about Kramer. He was simply too unpredictable.

Kramer, who apparently believed that Russo had already been chosen, began his letter innocently enough. He recalled asking Volberding months before to allow him to speak at the San Francisco conference, and noted that Volberding had "looked favorably upon my request." Kramer's letter continued:

I did not expect to be turned over to a committee of gay Uncle Toms, led by Dr. Wachter and Mr. Van Gorder.

As the founder of ACT UP, of which there are now a great many active chapters around the country, and the cofounder of Gay Men's Health Crisis—the two most important AIDS organizations in the country—I believe I am entitled to a little more respect than I have experienced with these two [men], culminating in my request being denied.

I think you will find it to prove a big mistake not to have honored my fervent solicitations. By snubbing me in such a fashion you have slapped in the face not only me and what I have stood for these past nine years, but every other AIDS activist. I trust that with the publication and circulation of this letter, ACT UPs everywhere will now commence their planning to join my call to action—at the conference—to let you, your committee, your conference, and the world that is watching know that, once again, an attempt has been made to silence us.

It is constantly amazing to me how often—when the offer is made, the hand extended, by those of us on another side of this battle, to cooperate—the chance to work in tandem is so casually and carelessly rejected.

Vito Russo, my good friend, who was chosen, was never consulted by your people, and, indeed, as your committee was informed, is not even interested in speaking, preferring that I do it. The fact that none of your people even bothered to talk to him is further proof that you are afraid of what I might say, which is greatly troubling.

Everyone had hoped that your conference, of all conferences, and in your city, of all cities, would allow the chance for divergent opinions to be aired publicly. Evidently such is not to be the case; and once again we face a conference homogenized, made bland, and blanched of open discussion of the many divisive issues that prevent AIDS from being cured.

I can assure you that you will now find it will be a conference otherwise. You have, in effect, thrown down the gauntlet, and I intend to see that it is taken up.

If you wish to view this letter as a threat, please do so.

All of us got a good chuckle over Kramer's "gay Uncle Toms." Dana, who is gay, walked into my office, extended his hand and said, "Hey, brother." My office staff, for a brief period, took to calling me "Tom." But our jocularity camouflaged the anxiety we shared.

I discussed the letter with Volberding, who counseled calm. "Larry has been sending off histrionic diatribes like this for the entire decade. They mean absolutely nothing," he said. He went on to say that, although Kramer did start GMHC and ACT UP, his present place in their leaderships was tenuous. "Even the activists find him to be an uncontrollable force."

Later that day, Dana called Kramer at home. Kramer harangued Dana about the issues laid out in the letter. However, one thing surprised Dana. In the middle of Kramer's ranting, Dana slipped in, "By the way, Bob isn't gay." Kramer, derailed for a moment, said, "Oh, I'm sorry," in a voice Dana described as sincerely apologetic. Dana also spoke to Vito Russo, informing him that, yes, he was on the short list of speakers for the opening ceremony, but that no final decision had been made. Russo told Dana that he was more than willing to speak if given the opportunity.

We heard nothing from Larry Kramer through the rest of December. On January 3, 1990, the *New York Times* carried a prominent article entitled "Rash, Rude and Effective, ACT UP Helps Change AIDS Policy." Kramer's role as founder and "elder statesman" of ACT UP was acknowledged and praised. Kramer's picture topped the piece; his piercing eyes were staring at me when the phone rang. "Larry Kramer," my secretary announced. I braced myself for the onslaught. After a very polite hello, he asked me when the opening ceremony program would be finalized. I gave him my standard answer that it would be decided sometime in the next couple of weeks, "after the committees meet."

"Exactly who are these committees?" he said. I ticked off a few lists, not divulging that this decision would be mine. "Well, I still feel like I should be the one to speak up there," he said. "Did you see me in the *Times*?!"

So that's what this was about, I thought. He's been given the blessing of the *New York Times*, and feels that his mantle has now been elevated to that of ACT UP's sage. His claim to be the one person capable of representing the activist perspective was now chiseled into the nation's most authoritative tablet.

"I can't think of anyone who will make a more effective speech," he continued.

"Larry," I said, "I'm very sympathetic. But your letter certainly didn't help any. We've got to take this thing to our committees, and even though they're perfectly ready to have the activist perspective represented at the opening ceremony, they may read the letter and say, 'Can we afford to take this kind of chance?' "

"I know it's not the first time that I've shot myself in the foot. The letter was written in great anger," he said. "I still think I'm the person to do it."

He went on to suggest a panel session on the politics of the epidemic—and how community activism can influence the politics. "It'll sort of be a session on starting an ACT UP in your neighborhood," he chuckled. He then ticked off a number of speakers both from in and outside of ACT UP who could represent the activist perspective. When I told Larry that I liked his idea quite a bit, he quickly added that he hoped I would not "take this as an alternative to me speaking in the opening. I'd be more than happy to do both."

I was frank. "I hope it's no surprise to you that you've got strong supporters, but also some opponents out there," I said. "Even when we talk to people in ACT UP, they often suggest other names to speak at the conference."

"Well, you have to realize," he said, "that ACT UP is a very peculiar animal. When someone has the energy to do something, we usually let them do it. I know the people you've been talking to, and they're not the right people to give you good information. They just happened to be the ones who volunteered to do this job. I don't think I've ever made a speech in public which has not been effective," he continued. "I want to be the one who gets this stuff on television. I feel that I've earned it."

The conversation gravitated to other matters. I asked him whether he ever worried that ACT UP would get too respectable. Could he see a day when ACT UP members would put on ties to sit on committees, or when the organization itself would become bureaucratized? Already, there were ACT UPs in forty U.S. cities and a smattering of other countries.

"There is that danger," he said. "We now have seats on the three biggest committees of the NIH, and we were asked this week to sit on another one by the CDC. I may be getting too soft in my old age, but I figure that you can't just scream and yell—you can't protest to get access to decision-making committees, and then not take part in the committees when you're asked. Maybe I am getting old."

We ended up the conversation back where we started—on the opening ceremony. "Larry, your letter made us worried that you might just express uncontrolled rage up there, and I don't think that would do anyone any good. The audience, as you know, is skeptically sympathetic. You lose them if you scream at them." He said that he understood that, and would give a moving speech suitable for the audience of scientists, clinicians, and HIV-infected people. "Would it make you feel better if I gave you my speech in advance and you could approve it?" he asked. I told him that I wasn't sure that he would want to do that, since it might be seen as censorship by his constituents. But this was only part of the story. I was truly concerned that this person—who flipped from wild activist to charming raconteur—could not be trusted. What guarantee would we have that the speech he had written a month prior to the conference would be the one that he would deliver in front of a worldwide audience?

However, I must admit that I was swayed by his charm. I walked into John Ziegler's office, and told him that I was reconsidering—that Kramer might be an appropriate, although risky, choice to speak in the opening ceremony. He had all the right credentials, he is widely acclaimed as a moving speaker, and he certainly wanted the part. "Well, let's think about it," John said. "If we pick him, we need to make it clear that he has to help us control ACT UP at the conference."

"That smacks a bit of 'arms for the Ayatollah' to me, John," I said.

"Yeah, but we're in the trenches now," he said, sighing. "This is the Middle East."

Dana brought me back to my senses a few minutes later. I told him of my conversation with Kramer, and that I was reconsidering using him in the opening. Dana was flabbergasted. "No way," he said. "He'd be great unless he's pissed off that day, and then we'd get it with both barrels. Don't you know that you should never negotiate with terrorists?"

That comment hit pay dirt. Although I had told Kramer that his letter had hurt his chance to be chosen, in actuality it had killed it. Since he had sent carbon copies of the letter to the press, a decision to invite Kramer to speak at the opening now would be seen as a capitulation to his threats of disruption. So, in fact, it was Kramer himself who had thrown down the gauntlet, and there was no way for us to pick it up.

Although Kramer's threats had, for practical purposes, excluded him from consideration as an opening ceremony speaker, there is little question that threats—often unstated —do influence decision-makers. "Though I admit I'm bothered by some of the intimidation, we need to have a partnership with them," Paul Volberding told the *Examiner*. And Dr. Anthony Fauci, Director of the National Institute of Allergy and Infectious Diseases at the National Institutes of Health, agreed. "We need to work with these people. They are intelligent, gifted, articulate people coming up with good, creative ideas."

Although it is these ideas—the thoughtfulness of many ACT UP proposals—that eventually impress many longtime ACT UP watchers like Fauci, our major interest was to avoid the disruption they might bring to the conference. This placed us in a precarious position: How could we avoid disruption but still produce a meaningful conference that did not shy away from controversial issues?

For the most part, we chose to invite the best speakers, even if they were unpopular among the *enfants terribles* of the epidemic. ACT UP blamed researchers like Dr. Dan Hoth, Director of NIH's Division of AIDS, and Dr. Margaret Fischl,

Director of AIDS at the University of Miami, for the slow pace of drug development. We felt they were the two best people to give an overview of clinical trials in AIDS (Hoth), and early treatment of HIV infection (Fischl). And so we invited them, knowing that we might also be inviting pandemonium.

On the other hand, when all else was equal between two speakers, we sometimes chose the one who would not provoke the activists. We were not particularly proud of these choices, but rationalized them by telling ourselves that we were looking after the greater good—producing a conference in which people could effectively share information. Gratuitous shouting and possible violence would help no one.

The case of Dr. Woodrow Myers, newly appointed New York City Health Commissioner, comes to mind. Myers, a black M.D., M.B.A., member of the first Presidential Commission on AIDS, and former Indiana Health Commissioner, was targeted by ACT UP for advocating a policy in which public health officials record the names of people infected with HIV. The policy, which has been implemented in other states, is favored by some public health officials as a means of tracking HIV-infected people to offer them early therapy and to counsel their sexual or drug-using contacts. Many activists (and other public health officials) criticize the strategy, contending that it is intrusive, discriminatory, and wasteful of precious public health dollars.

In October 1989, ten months before our conference and two months after Montreal, Dr. Stephen Joseph, Myers's predecessor as New York City Health Commissioner and the recipient of an ACT UP "zap" in Montreal, had been invited to address a smaller conference in San Francisco, the National AIDS Update. According to a letter Joseph would later write to San Francisco Health Director David Werdegar, one of the AIDS Update's organizers, Joseph was called by one of Update's staff and told that "due to threats of disruption by ACT UP if I appeared at the meeting, you wished me to

withdraw as a speaker. I of course refused to do so, and was
then informed . . . that you were 'changing the panel topic,'
and disinviting me as a speaker."

Joseph's letter continued:

> Beyond the issues of the importance of full and open
> debate to public health and medical care policy, I am
> most saddened by what I view as a step you have taken
> to vastly increase the likelihood of next June's Inter-
> national AIDS Conference in San Francisco becoming
> a pseudopolitical circus, rather than a scientific meet-
> ing.
>
> I regret that you have opted for appeasement of the
> loudest shouters rather than for the open airing of
> views: It is a strategy that very seldom works, and will
> not in this case.

Joseph's passionate letter caused us to reflect deeply on our
program philosophy. Were we appeasing the loudest shout-
ers? Or were we planning the best meeting for the most people? To this day, I am unsure. In any case, Woodrow Myers
was not asked to speak at the Sixth International Conference
on AIDS. And neither was Stephen Joseph.

As we had learned from our efforts on the immigration
issue, often the best approach was to work collaboratively
with the activists. Increasingly, as scientists recognized the
power of groups like ACT UP to mobilize the system, they
began to try to enlist the activists in their own causes. At one
meeting of the Community Task Force, Mark Jacobson, a
young AIDS physician and researcher at San Francisco General Hospital and a member of the Task Force, handed out
a memo that had been distributed in the AIDS clinic at the
hospital. The memo discussed federal guidelines that provided
for government reimbursement for AZT treatment only in

those HIV-infected people with T-helper cell counts below 200. (T-helper cells, also known as CD4 cells, are critical to the human immune system. Uninfected people have over 1,000 T-helper cells in each cubic milliliter of their blood.) Recent studies conducted by Doctors Volberding and Fischl had clearly demonstrated that patients with T-helper cell counts of less than 500 benefitted from use of AZT. But until the federal guidelines changed, read the memo, "patients with prescriptions for AZT who have between 200 and 500 CD4 cells will have their paperwork held. Once the guidelines are modified, we will contact the patients to pick up their AZT."

That such a memo existed, or even that a concerned physician chose to discuss it at the Community Task Force meeting was not remarkable. What was extraordinary was that Jacobson was asking for the "help" of the Task Force in effecting changes in government policy. "We can't provide AZT to our indigent patients who don't meet these criteria," he said. "We'll have to turn people away because there is no money. If the people around this table can do what it takes to raise consciousness or make a news story out of this, we can save lives."

Jacobson's plea reminded me of a conversation I had with an official of the American Lung Association at a meeting in Annapolis, Maryland. The official told me of the association's upcoming Boston conference on tuberculosis, a classic lung infection seen with increased frequency in AIDS patients. "We don't get enough press coverage at these conferences," he lamented. "One full day of the conference deals with tuberculosis and AIDS. Do you think we should talk to the activists to get them interested? If they're there, that'll get us some press, won't it?"

Both these examples demonstrate a recognition by those in the scientific community that the activists may have more power to change the medical system than do the scientists. As with all unharnessed sources of power, the strength of the activists can be used for good or evil. The doctor's suggestion that the activists get involved in AZT funding for indigent patients made sense, recognizing as it did the highly political nature of government resource allocation decisions. This of course begs the question of what happens to other individuals or groups whose causes are equally worthy of funding but who lack the loud voices of activists working on their behalf.

However, the Lung Association official had a different purpose in mind. He hoped to use the presence of activists to increase the press coverage of his event and gain greater visibility. I declined to help. First of all, I told him, my perception of Montreal was that many activists were there *because* the press was there, not vice versa. Furthermore, I told him that I thought he was playing with fire. Not only are the activists unpredictable (as they need to be in order to be effective), but they are proudly antiestablishment. Were they to sense that an administrator was trying to use their presence to gain increased visibility for his event, it would backfire. I told him that a reasonable guiding principle would be that if the activists take an interest in you, it would be wise to take an interest in them and begin constructive discussions to find out what they want. However, if they don't take an interest, it's probably best to leave well enough alone.

It might be like playing with fire, but the temptation to try to co-opt even the angriest activist is, at times, irresistible. Perhaps they stir within us a fantasy of operating in a world without constraints. As wary as I was of Larry Kramer, one day I asked him why ACT UP had not agitated over the immigration restrictions on people with HIV. Most of our help in fighting the Immigration Service had come from traditional AIDS lobbies such as Washington's AIDS Action Council. Scarcely a word of protest had been heard from ACT UP.

"It's just not an issue that has excited ACT UP," Kramer told me in October 1989, soon after I met him in New York. "A guy from Norway came to our meeting to talk about it, and we had to brush him off because there were so many other things higher on the list. Just this week we heckled Cuomo at the state legislature, and protested at Dinkins's inauguration. It's the local issues that tend to get us riled up."

I told him the conference remained concerned about the problem, and that we were still trying to change the Immigration Service policy. Like Dr. Jacobson and the Lung Association official, I asked Kramer for his help.

"I seem to be the repository for everybody who's got a problem in New York." He laughed. "A guy called me the other day. He said he'd been at a party at some nightclub, and there was unsafe sex going on and drugs being used during the party. He asked me to look into it. What the hell am I supposed to do?" He concluded by telling me that he'd try to get ACT UP more involved in the travel issue, but he wasn't sure that it would work.

Two days later, I told my wife of my discussion with Larry Kramer. Sure I knew it was chancy, but unlike the hapless officer of the Lung Association, I was sure ACT UP was going to be around during the conference. So why not try to involve them in something useful? "So I asked Kramer to try to get ACT UP interested in the travel issue," I said innocently.

"You did what?!" She gasped. "I can see it now—they'll be splashing red paint on Dick Thornburgh saying that Bob Wachter sent us."

"I never told them to go wild. I just told them that they might want to look into the issue," I retorted lamely.

"*Are you crazy?!*" She was exasperated. "What do you think he's going to do? Organize a letter-writing campaign?"

Although a letter-writing campaign might be an absurdity for ACT UP, much of the political movement on AIDS has come from advocacy groups treading more traditional paths. The combination of spirited protests by activist groups and behind-the-scenes lobbying by groups like the AIDS Action Council and the National Gay and Lesbian Task Force resulted in an unprecedented government response to the epidemic.

By 1989, in fact, the AIDS community began to confront a question born of its success: Was AIDS getting more than its fair share?

For the first time, some criticized AIDS funding as too generous when compared to the funding provided to fight other serious illnesses. For example, federal spending for AIDS reached $1.6 billion in 1990, a year after 40,000 Americans had died of the disease. At the same time, federal spending for cancer, which killed 500,000 in 1989, was $1.5 billion, and spending for heart disease, which killed 750,000, was less than $1 billion.

During the first five years of the AIDS epidemic, advocates for people with cancer and heart disease continued their quiet lobbying, while AIDS advocates eschewed political activism. Everyone who watched the epidemic unfold and witnessed the government's anemic response learned about a fundamental principle of American research: The system of funding is an inherently political process.

The metamorphosis in the second half of the 1980s was the recognition by AIDS advocates of this fundamental principle. Jeff Levi, then Executive Director of the National Gay and Lesbian Task Force, noted the transformation as early as 1985. "We have started to act like a traditional minority group," Levi said. "What AIDS has done is teach gays that the government has a positive contribution to make." Five years later, Levi would look back with pride: "Long after AIDS is gone, we will have changed how research is done in this country."

In 1989, three areas came under increased scrutiny. First, with AIDS claiming a larger and larger percentage of a fixed medical research pie, many began to question the equity of allocation. "AIDS has generated attention all out of proportion to other diseases," said Joel Hay, a health economist and senior research fellow at Stanford University's Hoover Institution. "It's new. It's fatal. It's associated with high-risk behavior. But if they had a quilt for victims of heart disease [like the famed AIDS Quilt], it would cover Washington, D.C., in two months."

AIDS advocates found themselves defending their budget requests against increasingly pointed attacks. Jean McGuire, Executive Director of the AIDS Action Council, recalled her testimony before Senator Thomas Harkin's appropriations subcommittee. "He interrupted me about two minutes into my talk and said, 'Now, Ms. McGuire, don't you think AIDS has claimed enough of the research budget?' And this is a congressman who's friendly to our cause."

The resistance encountered by AIDS advocates was predictable. The continuous push for more—resources, vigor, attention—though understandable, was destined to butt heads with the existence of other compelling resource needs. Economists have dispassionately described those who fail to recognize the scarcity of resources relative to wants as possessing a "romantic point of view." "The fact that we are constantly being confronted with the need to choose is attributed to capitalism, communism, advertising, the unions, war, unemployment, or any other convenient scapegoat," wrote Stanford health economist Victor Fuchs in his superb book, *Who Shall Live?* "Because *some* of the barriers to greater output and want satisfaction are clearly man-made, the romantic is misled into confusing the real world with the Garden of Eden. Because it denies the *inevitability* of choice, the romantic point of view is impotent to deal with the basic economic problems that face every society."

AIDS advocates were quick to point out that AIDS resources often "did not come at the expense of other health care needs." But this point of view is naive. Even if money did not directly translocate from a column entitled "diabetes research" to one entitled "AIDS research," the overall health care research pie remained essentially fixed; money spent on AIDS was money not spent on something else. Similarly, manpower hours used in expediting drug trials and grant reviews were not in limitless supply; it may be reasonably argued that their deployment in the cause of AIDS slowed important work in other areas. This is neither "wrong" nor "right" in any absolute sense of the words. The allocation of resources is a complex process involving value judgments and social choice.

The AIDS advocacy community shunned such economic analyses, and was correct in doing so. The advocate's job is not to understand society's perspective (that is not quite so, since often such understanding is crucial to effective advocacy), but to further his or her own agenda. The AIDS community had, in the last half of the 1980s, performed this job with unprecedented skill. But it was inevitable that others would eventually learn the game and begin to proffer effective counterpoints. And it was just as inevitable that policymakers, charged with protecting the whole of society's interests, would listen.

The second area cited by critics of AIDS advocacy was the change in the drug approval process. Although AIDS advocates were not the first to recognize the political nature of the process, they learned to influence it to a degree unmatched by any other disease lobby. When testing of new AIDS drugs proceeded too slowly, community groups like San Francisco's Project Inform began underground tests, directly challenging the FDA's regulatory authority. Meanwhile, ACT UP conducted massive protests at FDA headquarters, and threatened to sabotage government-sponsored drug trials. The result: an expedited drug approval process hailed as lifesaving by AIDS advocates, but criticized as risky and inequitable by others. AZT, for example, won FDA approval in less than four months, compared with the usual two-year waiting period. James Todd, Senior Vice President of the American Medical Association, took note of the AZT approval and said, "It's distorted all the traditional principles of drug approval. Penicillin couldn't get through that fast."

Finally, critics of the AIDS lobby pointed to the lobby's emphasis on developing and testing new drugs to treat those already infected by HIV, as opposed to prevention programs. Politically, this bias can be explained by the lobby's genesis in gay activism of the 1970s. Gay men were by far the majority of people initially infected by HIV, and the relatively educated population quickly learned to practice prevention. By 1985, the risk of an uninfected gay man in San Francisco becoming infected with HIV dropped to almost nil. Despite some recent reports of recidivism, many AIDS activists agree with Michael Nesline of ACT UP, who said: "We're fighting for people for whom the question of prevention is a moot point."

The concentration on finding a cure left other groups still at risk for HIV—primarily heterosexual blacks and Hispanics of the urban ghettoes on the east and west coasts—uneducated and unprotected. Although representatives of these communities have made small inroads among the lobbyists and activists, the AIDS political machine was and remains overwhelmingly gay. The focus on cure also rendered the activist agenda irrelevant to the staggering problems of Africa and other countries in the developing world, where the average annual per capita health care budget of less than five dollars makes the superiority of one antiviral agent over another cruelly immaterial. For these countries, prevention is the only reasonable strategy.

AIDS advocates defend the priority given to AIDS in recent years. AIDS is different, they say, because it is epidemic and infectious. It also strikes all ages, whereas cancer and heart disease tend to strike mostly people in their fifties and sixties. Prompt action could contain the spread of the causative agent, which is not the case in cancer or heart disease. In addition, AIDS has struck overwhelmingly in a dozen urban centers around the country, bringing the public health system in these cities to its knees.

Perhaps the most cogent argument for treating AIDS differently from other diseases is the bang-for-the-buck theory:

After decades of research on cancer and heart disease at a cost of billions of dollars, there has been incremental progress, but nothing resembling a cure. And it is unlikely that another billion would eradicate these diseases. On the other hand, another billion dollars spent on AIDS could lead to a pivotal advance—perhaps even a cure. Although unlikely, this scenario's possibility explains the activists' crusade for a "Manhattan Project" for AIDS.

In the final analysis, it may be that some of the criticism of the AIDS lobby was born of jealousy—as advocates of other health care causes saw that AIDS had come in just a few years to dominate the research agenda of a nation. They now realized what the AIDS advocates had long recognized: The medical research establishment in the United States is divided into disease-oriented fiefdoms, and each fiefdom is considerably better at asking for money for its cause than looking at the big picture and setting global priorities. That politics might decide something as important as funding for research and prevention of AIDS and other deadly diseases should come as no surprise. After all, it's the American way.

As the 1980s ended, the AIDS lobby began to hit some brick walls. First, it began to feel the backlash of the non-AIDS research and advocacy communities, who entered the political fray and lodged effective arguments for bigger slices of the pie for Alzheimer's, cancer, and heart disease. Second, many of the early gains in AIDS had come from generally sympathetic scientists within the Public Health Service, who had the power to modify the regulatory process or redistribute funds under their control. Having exhausted that option, most of the sought-after funds were now controlled by hard-nosed administration bureaucrats, not nearly as sympathetic to the cause as the scientists, and not as accessible to lobbying efforts. To quench the continued thirst of the activists now required a larger pie—a pie not readily available in a climate of deficit reduction. And so we had a recipe for frustration.

AIDS protests, even ACT UP's most spirited efforts, had always been characterized by nonviolence. But as the community grew more desperate, we began to worry. Was there more than bluster in Larry Kramer's threats? Might all this anger eventually explode? If so, were we sitting on the powder keg?

Our fear of violence at the conference was not mere paranoia. After all, the conference was scheduled for the same week as Gay and Lesbian Freedom Week. Jim Foster's "eight-hundred-pound gorilla" would bring some quarter of a million gays to the streets of San Francisco during the conference. In fact, the week would culminate with the Gay and Lesbian Freedom Day Parade, scheduled to start at precisely the same time as the conference's closing ceremony.

I began to have nightmares—vivid ones—in which column after column of parade-goers made the left turn at Third and Market and moved en masse toward the Moscone Center's glass front doors. Hundreds of police on horseback were waiting for them, but the ACT UPers who had succeeded in diverting the parade rushed the crowd forward, a human battering ram. Like a scene out of *Gandhi*, the police raised their billy clubs to stave off the angry mob and. . . . At that point, I would wake up, drenched in sweat.

To prevent this scenario, I knew, would take more than beefed-up security. The activists needed to feel that the conference was *theirs*—that their aspirations and frustrations were given voice in the program. How to do this, while still preserving the scientific integrity of the meeting, was unclear. I needed some advice.

I spoke to Dr. Mervyn Silverman, President of the American Foundation for AIDS Research (AmFAR), one of the conference's cosponsors. "We need to convince the activists of the value of the conference," Silverman said. "The exchange of information, and even more importantly, the international focus on AIDS for the week, are indispensable to the global fight against the epidemic." I told him that I agreed, but could understand the perspective of those angry at the conference and the scientists. After all, the community was being ravaged.

"What I've discovered in this epidemic," Silverman said, "is that there is absolutely nothing that's simple. When you think you have the thing figured out, and you've considered every possible angle, you'll always find someone on the other side. Even the easy ones come back at you." Silverman, who as San Francisco's Health Director in the early 1980s was at the epicenter of the controversy surrounding the closing of the gay bathhouses, spoke from experience. "I found that when you are hearing all these different perspectives," he continued, "what you need to do is sit across the table and take the other guy's perspective for a while. After you've done that, and only after you've done that, can you say to those you disagree with that you can't do what they want."

Silverman's wisdom convinced me to return to the Community Task Force to solicit more recommendations about the conference program, especially the opening ceremony. But we needed to do more. After Montreal, we needed to convince the activists of the value of the conference. As with so many other answers, this one came from Jonathan Mann, Director of the World Health Organization's Global Programme on AIDS and arguably the single most effective person in the international AIDS sphere.

Mann began working in the public health field in 1975, after earning his M.D. at Washington University in St. Louis. For the next decade, he served as Chief Medical Officer for the State of New Mexico, a position not generally looked upon as a stepping-stone to preeminence. Then in 1984 Mann moved to Africa, to head the Centers for Disease Control's AIDS program in Zaire, a nation devastated by "slim disease."

In 1986, he was summoned to Geneva, Switzerland, to develop a "Global Programme on AIDS" (GPA) for the World

Health Organization. He was given a budget of $500,000 and a staff of one. Mann remembered having been impressed by a nurse he met at a small AIDS conference in 1985, and asked this nurse, Kathleen Kay, to leave her hometown of Woy Woy, Australia, to join him in Geneva. She jumped at the opportunity, and the two (along with social scientist Manuel Carballo of Gibraltar and public health expert Daniel Tarantola of France) began to build the fledgling program from scratch.

Between 1986 and 1989, the team built the GPA into the largest program in WHO history. Despite operating in an environment of international hostility and suspicion, under Mann's leadership GPA concluded agreements to establish AIDS programs in 155 countries. The staff grew to 220 members in Geneva alone, and the yearly budget to $109 million. June Osborn, Dean of the School of Public Health at the University of Michigan and Chair of the U.S. National Commission on AIDS, said of Mann: "From July 1986 when he didn't even have an office, to more than a hundred and fifty usable, constructive agreements on such a sensitive issue is the most brilliant job of international creative work that I know of."

Much of Mann's success is attributed to his personal charisma, which is self-evident and genuine. His boundless energy, though, was what impressed me most. Kathleen Kay described physicians and researchers who came to Geneva to work with GPA. "Many would come expecting to have a fairly pleasant stay in Europe," Kathleen told me, "with trips to Paris every few weeks. But the pace at the Global Programme is intense, and there is no time for play."

Mann drove himself to meet lofty standards, and expected the same from his staff. Kathleen was scheduled to attend a meeting in Montreal three days after the closing of the Fifth International Conference, also in Montreal. When the conference ended, Mann sent her back to the office in Geneva to work. "There are three good work days before your next meeting," he told her. Kathleen was incredulous, since those three "work days" were Saturday, Sunday, and Monday. But she returned and worked.

Since WHO, like Silverman's AmFAR, was a conference cosponsor, Mann attended our International Steering Committee meeting in late fall, 1989. He shared our fear of disruption and violence at the conference. We listened intensely.

"The activists don't recognize how much they turn off people from developing countries attending the conference," Mann said. "The level of activism and the informality among Americans is totally foreign to people in developing countries. For many, the Montreal conference was their only source of information related to AIDS. They were there to take notes. When the disruptions began, not only were they surprised by them, but they were hurt by them."

We all recalled the speech in Montreal by Dame Nita Barrow, Barbados's delegate to the United Nations. Barrow spoke poignantly about the impact of AIDS on her country, describing one village in which an elderly woman was left to raise twelve grandchildren after her own six children died of AIDS. Her offspring were buried in neat graves behind her house, because the local church refused to bury their ravaged bodies in its graveyard. Barrow concluded her moving story by pleading for compassion for "victims of this disease."

Randy Shilts, writing in *Mother Jones*, described the rest of the scene: "At this point, the ACT UP word police took up booing. Barrow had used the word 'victim', a major semantic no-no among AIDS activists. Unaware of her gaffe, Barrow used the word again when calling for compassion, only to be greeted with hisses. She looked curiously at the protestors: Were these people *against* compassion?"

The incident was only one of many that, Mann said, disturbed the visitors from developing countries. "I see the conference as an embassy in a foreign country," Mann said, "a place to which people in every country come to grow and share information. It should be an international zone, and those who disrupt it for their own local or national purposes should recognize that they are violating this international zone." The implication was clear: If the conference was an international zone like an embassy, those who would violate such a zone were terrorists.

"I don't really care what happens outside the conference walls because that is fair game for national and local politics to play out," Mann continued, his voice filled with emotion. "But I care deeply about what happens inside. Many people in developing countries say to me, 'Don't you think the conference has outlived its usefulness?' The answer, if the level of disruption remains high, may very well be yes."

Dana and I were convinced that our best hopes for the conference lay in getting this message to the activists. This was an area of vulnerability for them—as Kramer had said, it was hard to get them interested in international issues. If we could convince the activists that they were hurting AIDS efforts in developing countries by disrupting the conference, their sense of political correctness might moderate their demonstrations. We asked Mann to speak to the Community Task Force, our best conduit to the activist community.

Mann was fifteen minutes late to the Task Force meeting, having been delayed while visiting the Names Project, home of the AIDS Quilt. One of the Task Force members, a clergyman wearing his religious garb, came in as the conference room was filling up. He sat down and noticed that the chair next to him was unoccupied. He looked around, saw no Jonathan Mann, and said, "I guess we're still waiting for Himself."

Finally Mann entered, not exactly "Himself" but our best approximation. Treading carefully—expressing his concerns to the activists while not lecturing them—he spoke: "The meeting is a very precious thing. It is unprecedented in the history of any medical or health-related meetings, in that it is an international meeting in the truest sense of the word. People come from all over the world to share knowledge with each other and to learn what they need to know to save lives."

Mann went on to highlight the fragility of this participation. "I sense a real possibility that the international community will pull out of this meeting if it gets any more disruptive than it has been." Was he threatening to pull WHO out of the meetings? someone asked. "It's absolutely not a threat," he said gravely, "and should not be taken as such. I don't feel like I'm in a threatening mood. What I really feel is scared."

Mike Shriver from ACT UP told Mann of the Task Force's list of recommendations related to the conference program. "The chances of disruption will go down significantly if the conference listens to these recommendations," he said. I assured Shriver that we were following virtually all of the recommendations. But I was not reassured. To my mind, the level of disruption would have much more to do with the conference's role as the world's largest AIDS soapbox than any specifics related to program or logistics.

Paul Boneberg agreed that disruptions might be inevitable at the meeting. "There will always be a fundamental conflict between patients who empower themselves and their doctors." Therefore, Boneberg added, there was no way he could guarantee that there would be no disruptions.

"I am not looking for guarantees," Mann said sadly. "I know that I can't get any. I thought it was important that I tell you what I've been hearing around the world—to sensitize you to these issues. I also wanted to give myself an opportunity to truly understand your perspective."

I was impressed watching Mann as he listened to the activists, nodding his head in support of all they were saying. "Yes, I agree," he would say after Task Force members passionately argued against AIDS discrimination or in support of increased AIDS funding. From time to time he went beyond mere affirmation, putting himself in the sympathetic position of being as powerless as they were to effect changes in mistaken policies like the Immigration Service's position on travel by PWAs. "Yes, I know this is terrible," he would say. "What do you think we can do about it?" And then he listened to the reply and developed a plan to work together for change.

But passive assent alone could not win the respect of the members of the Task Force. Although there were some in the group too insecure to tolerate a challenge to their points of view by Dr. Mann, I identified Paul Boneberg as one person who would not only tolerate such a challenge, but gain respect for the challenger. Mann perceived this also and used it to his advantage.

Boneberg spoke passionately about the role of activists in combatting the epidemic. "Of course," he said, "everyone knows that the activists have been responsible for the majority of worldwide funding and public health efforts to fight AIDS, including in the developing countries."

Mann had been looking down at his long fingers, clasped together on the table. He looked up and stared at Boneberg. "No, I'm afraid that's wrong," he said matter-of-factly.

Boneberg finished speaking, and Mann spoke again. "I agree with virtually everything you've said, but I'm afraid I need to take exception to your statement that the activists are responsible for developing-country support." Mann cited the devastation wrought by AIDS in Africa, and increasingly in countries like India and Brazil. "The sum total of American support for fighting AIDS outside the U.S. is about thirty to forty million a year," he said. "That's not a number that I, or I think you, would think was adequate. Unfortunately, I don't think the activists have had any influence on prevention and care outside the United States." Paul Boneberg was unused to being challenged so directly. He nodded in agreement, and I never heard him make the same assertion again. Equally important, his respect for Mann blossomed.

Months later, after the immigration issue heated up and community groups took to criticizing the conference once again, an article appeared in the *Bay Area Reporter*, a leading San Francisco gay newspaper. "People from developing nations . . . get basically all their medical information each year from this conference," Paul Boneberg said. "So if these people come here and find the conference . . . disrupted to the point they cannot get information, how does this help us who are trying to stop this disease?" Jonathan Mann's words to the Community Task Force had taken root.

Afterwards, I drove Jonathan back to his hotel. He seemed pleased with the meeting, but remained frankly worried about the future of the conferences. "At some point," he said, "if the level of disruption grows, people will ask whether six million spent on this conference is the best way to spend AIDS money. Right now I have an answer—this conference is the major way that information is shared among the peoples of the world to fight the HIV epidemic. If things get any more disrupted, I will no longer be able to say this, and I expect the level of support for the meeting will decrease drastically." He paused for a moment, as if to reflect on the larger picture.

"I hope you realize that you're in the middle of something much bigger than just the International Conference on AIDS," he continued. "This whole situation—the relationship between the scientists and the activists, the relationship between domestic and international players, the political volatility of the issue—is unprecedented in the annals of any health-related issue."

My earlier innocence having long since passed, I nodded my head in weary, knowing agreement.

7 THE INVITATION LIST

Notwithstanding all our efforts to work with the activists and attend to the issues of the developing world, none of us doubted that the heart of the program was still the science. However, by late 1989, Ziegler, Volberding, and I were spending so much time forging coalitions and dousing political fires that many of the scientists on the Local Organizing Committee began to doubt our commitment to their cause. In defense of our concessions to the Task Force, we tried to explain what we had come to understand—that the relevance and universality of the conference depended on integrating the concerns of the community. But some scientists weren't buying. To them, we appealed to a sense of expediency: "In the present political climate, even if your goal is to put on the most research-oriented scientific meeting possible, you would still try to satisfy the activists."

Still, some scientists remained as skeptical of our efforts as the activists. We told them of our plans to be much more selective in choosing abstracts to increase the quality of the program. The afternoon basic science sessions would be at the Marriott Hotel, a block away from the Moscone Center, where we thought most of the commotion would be. We worked endlessly to improve the session logistics, so that the delegates would get the most out of presentations.

It was not until we received the review of our NIH conference grant application that we understood the depth of scientific skepticism. Jim Hill, Anthony Fauci's deputy director at the National Institute of Allergy and Infectious Diseases and a strong conference supporter, was trying to shepherd our grant through the NIH bureaucracy. "There are some folks at NIH who feel that this is not a scientific conference anymore, and therefore are reluctant to support it," Hill said. When we saw the actual review, we knew that Hill's use of the word "reluctant" was charitable. Through the whims of the NIH bureaucracy, the grant went to a basic science committee for review. The committee subjected us to five pages of vituperation:

"The AIDS pandemic is an important world health issue and it is unfortunate the plans for the scientific program for this key international meeting are not well-developed," read the review. "It is also unclear why the conference organizers have placed the important charge of program director in the hands of a recently-appointed clinical instructor." I'll live, I thought, and read on.

"The conference will be exceptionally well-covered by the press. . . . This meeting has the potential for informing the public, for increasing the awareness of how HIV-I and HIV-II spread and of the importance of compassionate care for those with AIDS. . . . However, this proposal does not appear to present a cohesive and timely scientific program, the central framework on which the Sixth International Conference on AIDS should rest."

The basic scientists on the NIH panel must have had chest pain thinking that the three main organizers—Ziegler, Volberding, and myself—were all primarily clinical, and not laboratory, researchers. Worst of all, my research interests also included medical ethics and health policy. "The seemingly inadequate nature of the scientific program for this meeting," the review concluded, "would appear to be based on the rather narrow focus on AIDS which these three individuals represent and their failure to go to the greater AIDS community to organize a strong and relevant program."

If the reviewers understood that our job was to structure the overall program and plan the logistics, and that decisions about scientific research would be made by a hundred-person basic science committee, headed by internationally respected researcher Jay Levy, they did not let on. Through the support of Hill, Fauci, and Jack Whitescarver in the NIH Office of AIDS Research, the grant was eventually funded. Our egos were a bit damaged, but what the hell—the conference needed the bucks.

Our efforts to placate the basic scientists had begun in earnest with the criticism leveled at the Montreal meeting by Dr. Robert Gallo of the National Cancer Institute. Gallo, the "co-discoverer" of the AIDS virus along with Luc Montagnier of the Pasteur Institute, was the loftiest of the AIDS superstars. If Gallo doesn't come to our meeting, we thought as we left Montreal, it will be hard to call the meeting a success.

Both Gallo and Montagnier had long histories with the International Conferences on AIDS. By the time of the Stockholm and Montreal gatherings, Gallo and Montagnier's side-by-side lectures had become conference ritual. Sure, Gallo's presentations were sometimes arrogant and Montagnier's English difficult to decipher, but these were the icons of the epidemic: the *co-discoverers of the virus*. The term was the yearly mantra uttered by each conference's chairman as he introduced the two great men.

Even though we thought it was important to have the support of Gallo and Montagnier, by 1989 many had begun to tire of the same well-worn speeches by the same scientists.

We considered the ultimate sacrilege: to invite neither Gallo nor Montagnier to lecture at one of the conference's main plenary sessions.

Jonathan Mann disagreed with us. Although he understood and agreed with our desire to inject new blood into the major sessions, he felt that Gallo and other scientific superstars would be looking for any excuse not to come to the meeting. Their absence, Mann thought, would become a major issue and a self-fulfilling prophecy, eventually leading to the demise of the International Conferences on AIDS.

Because their dispute over the discovery of HIV had taken an agreement between the Presidents of the United States and France to resolve, decisions about Gallo and Montagnier were matters of international diplomacy. If we invited Gallo to speak at the opening ceremony, we had to invite Montagnier as well, or risk an international incident. Furthermore, if Gallo and Montagnier were speaking, other luminaries of the epidemic such as James Curran of the CDC and Samuel Broder of the National Cancer Institute must also speak. Rather like a wedding—if we invite Harvey, then we have to invite *all* the second cousins—the conference's invitation list could quickly grow unwieldy.

After weeks of internal debate, we decided that there was only one way to move Gallo and Montagnier off the plenary session invitation list—by choosing no one to speak at a conference plenary session if they had given a plenary lecture at a past international AIDS conference. The virtues of this decision were soon apparent. It allowed us to elevate some younger researchers, often the ones who were actually doing the work rather than administering the lab or program, to the forefront of the epidemic. Moreover, the decision allowed us to remove Gallo and Montagnier from the plenary list without appearing to target them personally.

After our decision to deny Gallo and Montagnier their usual plenary showcases, we invited both to speak at smaller afternoon basic science sessions. Neither was particularly thrilled. Gallo asked to see which scientists were scheduled to speak in the plenary sessions before accepting our invitation. Montagnier felt that the fifteen minutes he was allocated for his talk was insufficient. "I have some important data to present, and if I am not able to do it, I might reconsider my participation in the conference," he wrote.

Montagnier did appear, and gave a controversial talk outlining his latest theory: that a class of simple microbes—called mycoplasmas—are important cofactors that may facilitate transition of the AIDS virus from asymptomatic infection to fatal illness. Montagnier's supportive evidence was scanty, and many scientists were unconvinced. The CDC's James Curran reportedly called the theory "nonsense."

Gallo, scheduled to speak on the last day of the conference, was the subject of hundreds of press inquiries. Beginning with the publication of a thirty-thousand-word Gallo exposé in the *Chicago Tribune* in November 1989, many journalists now questioned the Official History. Was Gallo really the "codiscoverer of HIV"? Or had he—either accidentally or intentionally—misappropriated a virus from Montagnier's lab and called it his own?

Like a scientific Donald Trump, Gallo, who once could do no wrong by the press, now could do no right. I sensed that the press was interested in Gallo's appearance not to praise him, but to pillory him. Under the circumstances, I understood why he might not wish to subject himself to further public flogging, and made plans to replace him if necessary. Still, he had not contacted me to cancel until the morning of his talk, when I received a letter from him.

"As you know," it began, "I have an unbroken record of attendance and participation in all the past International Conferences on AIDS. That is the measure of my appreciation of the importance of the conferences and the reason I want to fully explain my inability to attend this year's meeting in San Francisco."

Gallo went on to explain that Soviet President Gorbachev,

during a recent summit in Washington, had personally asked him to meet with Soviet scientists. This, Gallo said, would require a longer stay in Eastern Europe and the U.S.S.R. than originally planned, thus forcing him to cancel his conference appearance.

"It is important to me that my absence will not be misinterpreted or regarded in any way other than my commitment to improving international scientific relationships toward those goals we all share."

Some journalists, of course, did "misinterpret" Gallo's absence as an avoidance of their notebooks and kleig lights. Others commented that Gallo might be reacting to being stripped of his permanent plenary status. One month after the conference ended, Gallo called me.

"I've gotten some bad press on this," he said, "but that's not as important as preserving the relationship between one scientist and another." (He was clearly one scientist; I guessed that the other was me.) "People said that my missing the meeting was arrogance—because I wasn't a plenary speaker—but it wasn't that at all. I understood perfectly what you were doing, and it was right. When I give meetings, I never have the same person speak six years in a row. You need new blood."

He went on to describe his conversation with Gorbachev at the Washington, D.C., state dinner. "I just couldn't say no."

But he was clearly exasperated by all the press reaction. "People are always making more of things than they really are when it comes to me," he lamented.

I reassured him that the conference had gone well, despite his absence. In fact, things had changed drastically since Montreal. In June 1989, we were obsessed with trying to plan the kind of meeting that Robert Gallo would want to attend. By June 1990, Gallo the "co-discoverer" was merely a sideshow, a fallen icon trying desperately to mend the fabric of his reputation.

* * *

Just as the opening ceremony in Montreal had set the tone for that conference, I firmly believed that our opening ceremony would presage the outcome of our meeting. The scientists would want a demonstration of the scientific integrity of the conference, while the activists would want evidence of our commitment to their agenda. And, like a drunken crowd at a bullfight, many of the hundreds of journalists in attendance would be anticipating a good brawl.

By late 1989, we knew three people who would not speak in the opening ceremony: Larry Kramer, Robert Gallo, and Luc Montagnier. But it was time to decide who would speak. There were a few givens. Ziegler, Volberding, UCSF Chancellor Julius Krevans, San Francisco Mayor Art Agnos, and I would all deliver brief welcomes to the audience. June Osborn, the highly respected Chair of the U.S. National Commission on AIDS, would speak on "Science and Public Health." UCSF virologist Jay Levy, who had lived in the shadows of Gallo and Montagnier for years, would shine with an overview of basic science. And Jonathan Mann would provide a review of the grim state of the epidemic in the developing world.

For the keynote speech, we looked for someone who could speak to issues beyond the science and politics—someone who could touch the audience and help them consider a new perspective. Our first choice, holocaust survivor and Nobel Peace Prize winner Elie Wiesel, originally accepted our invitation to speak about AIDS as a modern holocaust. A few months later, he declined our invitation, citing scheduling problems. We wondered whether the threats of disruption had scared him away.

We considered a number of world figures to replace Wiesel, including Archbishop Desmond Tutu, Barbara Bush, Mother Teresa, the Dali Lama, and President Vaclav Havel of Czechoslovakia. All of these candidates, we feared, would flunk what I called the "press conference test." Even if they spoke about

AIDS, the questions at the press conference would likely be about their own political baggage and not the epidemic. At last, we turned to Eunice Kiereini, Chair of Family Health for the Foundation of Kenya, a soft-spoken and wonderfully eloquent Kenyan nurse-midwife who has thought deeply about the devastating effects on women and children wrought by AIDS as it has cut a wide swath across Africa. Kiereini accepted, providing us with a compelling and unassailable keynote speaker.

But we agonized over the roles of two major players in the ceremony: the activists and President George Bush. Once again, we turned to the members of the Community Task Force for counsel.

After the Montreal conference ended, we had received three letters that profoundly affected our plans for our opening ceremony. The first was written by Leon McKusick, the HIV-infected psychologist who would eventually cochair the Community Task Force. Leon wrote of our need to "convey to the community that the principal concern of the . . . conference is the end of the loss of human life, beyond considerations of politics, finance, and personal advancement." He suggested beginning the opening ceremony with a public show of grief for those lost to the epidemic, and urged that we choose an activist as a major opening ceremony speaker.

Pierre Ludington, the other HIV-infected member of the conference's Local Organizing Committee, while agreeing with McKusick about the need for an HIV-positive AIDS advocate in the ceremony, was concerned about providing a soapbox for an angry activist. "This person's personality, concerns, involvement, emphasis, and passion will set the tone for many people for the rest of the week. Also this person will be the example for the thousands of HIV-infected people who have no chance or no desire to be at the conference, but whose interests are paramount to having the conference— the people who live their lives with calm determination. . . .

I do not want to listen to an angry self-serving diatribe that serves an only ACT UP or activist-type agenda. There are people who can speak to many facets of the epidemic, who can teach us activism without posturing, who can highlight compassion that is real, and who can point to lives that are lived with dignity, but without activism, that are just as right and valuable as others we have come to listen to because they are too loud and empowered by what is fast becoming a self-perpetuating system. It is time to listen to others."

The final letter came from Ronald Stall, a medical anthropologist who works at UCSF's Center for AIDS Prevention Studies. Stall worried about the volatility of the conference's timing. "We have to recognize the fact that the conference is timed to coincide with the Lesbian and Gay Freedom Day Parade," he wrote. "This parade has historically attracted as many as 300,000 participants. The size of this year's parade will swell as a result of the understandable wish to use the conference as a stage for a show of force by a community under attack. This has created what seems to me to be a scary situation: There will be a lot of affected (and infected) people locked out of a conference that is about their survival and the survival of the people that they love. The closest analogy in American political history that I can think of is to the situation of Chicago in 1968."

Stall pleaded for us to depoliticize the opening ceremony. "I think the opening session of the conference should be used as a memorial service for San Franciscans who have died of AIDS," he wrote. "Inviting President Bush will only serve to inflame the anger. . . . Why not avoid the twin pitfalls of politics and boredom and use the conference to put a genuinely human face on our fellow citizens that we have lost to AIDS?"

These letters solidified our commitment to highlight the PWA and activist perspectives in the opening ceremony, but to do so in a way that moved, and did not scold, the audience. It was this commitment that, in the end, led us to reject

Larry Kramer as the activist speaker, instead choosing Leon McKusick, writer Vito Russo, and Sallie Perryman, a black woman who had been infected by her husband. McKusick, Dana, and a New York producer named Jane Rosette also filmed a moving video of a rainbow coalition of PWAs presenting their "Personal Perspectives on the Epidemic." We felt confident that we had given voice to the activist and the nonactivist PWA points of view. So far, so good.

Deciding what to do with President George Bush was going to be tougher.

On a warm, muggy evening in Georgetown in 1987, President Ronald Reagan gave his first major speech on AIDS on the eve of the Third International Conference on AIDS. The occasion was an AmFAR-sponsored $250-a-plate dinner, replete with the superstars of the entertainment, political, and AIDS worlds. Reagan's speech focussed mostly on calls for widespread compulsory AIDS testing—of immigrants, prison inmates, and couples seeking marriage licenses. He paid little attention to prevention strategies, access to care, or the federal research effort.

George Bush, then Vice President, spoke the next day at the opening ceremony of the conference. The lineup for that ceremony speaks legions about the political changes in AIDS that would occur over the next three years. Appearing with Bush were Assistant U.S. Secretary of Health Robert Windom, Deputy Assistant Secretary for Health Lowell Harmison, Carlyle Guerra de Macedo, Director of the Pan-American Health Organization, and C. Everett Koop, U.S. Surgeon General. If the organizers of the Washington conference had been pressured to highlight the PWA perspective in the opening, there was no evidence that they acceded.

Bush's speech, like Reagan's, was long on compulsory testing, short on other strategies most public health experts consider more useful. Unlike Reagan, who had chosen the rarified atmosphere of the Georgetown dinner party for his "coming out," Bush was roundly heckled by the activists scattered among the crowd of five thousand conference delegates at the Washington Hilton. In contrast, Surgeon General Koop, who opposed mandatory testing and favored information campaigns to stem the AIDS tide, was given a standing ovation. At one point, puzzled by the audience reaction, Bush turned to an aide and asked, "Are those the homosexuals?" The comment was recorded by a live microphone.

As we deliberated over inviting President Bush, we thought it was unlikely that he and his handlers had forgotten that reception. ACT UP had not even been born at the time of the Washington Conference. The group's presence in large numbers at our conference would make the President even less likely to accept an invitation.

On the other hand, there were some clues that Bush might agree to speak in San Francisco. Unlike his predecessor as President, Bush seemed to be genuinely concerned about the plight of PWAs. He favored the passage of one bill banning AIDS discrimination in the workplace and another mandating harsh penalties for hate crimes against gays. During a visit to the NIH to see adults and children with AIDS, Bush called for "compassion and understanding" for people with the disease. "Incredibly," the President said, "some are still afraid of holding an AIDS patient because they're afraid of getting AIDS." He then hugged and kissed several of the children to demonstrate his point.

Precedent also increased the chance of a Bush acceptance. After the appearance in Stockholm by Swedish Prime Minister Ingvar Carlsson and in Montreal by Canadian Prime Minister Brian Mulroney, Bush would take a political gamble in declining our invitation. Finally, the increase in the size and importance of the conference, we thought, would render a "no" answer more politically risky to the President.

As we weighed the likelihood of a Bush acceptance or rejection, we had not considered the possibility of a third course—that Bush might do what Reagan had done and ask his Vice President to stand in for him—until one meeting of the Local Organizing Committee. "Don't forget," said conference fundraiser Dennis Hartzell, "he could always give us the Bird."

We all looked askance for a moment, but then deciphered Hartzell's reference. Bush might suggest his Vice President, conservative Dan Quayle, as a stand-in, especially if he wished to demonstrate to the Republican right wing that he was unbowed by the activists. Since Quayle is by turns ignored and reviled by the gay and AIDS communities, his selection would be seen as a direct slap in the face.

I met with George Galasso, who served as chair of the 1987 Washington conference and now directs extramural research at the NIH. I told Galasso that we were inclined to invite Bush to the opening, and Secretary of Health and Human Services Louis Sullivan to the closing ceremony. "Quayle would be an extraordinarily unpopular choice in San Francisco," I told him. "I'm worried that we'll invite Bush, but then get a call from the White House suggesting that we invite Quayle in his stead." I asked him whether he had received such a call when he invited President Reagan but ended up with Vice President Bush at the opening ceremony of the Washington Conference. His answer was not reassuring.

"We invited the President," Galasso said. "A few weeks later, we got back a letter telling us that the President would be unable to attend, but that the Vice President *would* be speaking in his place."

The fear of being "given the Bird" was not the only reason that we hesitated with our invitation to George Bush. A Bush appearance would be a logistical and security nightmare. Secret Service officers, acutely aware of Mulroney's experience in Montreal where there had been no metal detector, and no weapon or bomb search, would insist on clearing the Moscone Center at least an hour before a Bush speech to go over the venue with a fine-tooth comb. The Secret Service knew that the Royal Canadian Mounted Police had held Mulroney backstage and, with ACT UP sitting front and center in the VIP seats, had recommended against his taking the podium. The decision to speak was made by Mulroney himself, and though he kept a stiff upper lip during his speech, it was the perspiring lip of a fearful man. The Secret Service would ensure no repetition of this scene during a Bush appearance at the Moscone Center, but the price tag in terms of dollars, convenience, and ambience would be high.

Moreover, Mr. Bush's presence would flunk the "press conference test" in a major way. His visit to San Francisco would be a lightning rod for major demonstrations, only some of which would pertain to AIDS. With ACT UP already coming to the party, did we really need battles over South Africa, abortion, and acid rain? At its best, a Bush visit would distract from the major goal of the conference, the dissemination of scientific information related to AIDS.

Despite the likelihood of a decline from Bush, I still favored making the offer. If the President was not at the meeting because of our failure to invite him, the heat would be directed at us. But if he chose to say no to our invitation, the onus would be on him. One could almost hear the echoes of Ted Kennedy's famous "Where is George?" gathering in the distance. I also favored the invitation because it would give the President a forum for a major policy address, one he might take up if he had something consequential to say about the epidemic.

The issue was complex and important enough to be raised at the monthly meeting of the Local Organizing Committee. I began the discussion by listing what I saw to be the pros and cons of the Bush invitation.

The discussion was lively and passionate. Most of the scientists felt strongly that Bush's presence should be discouraged, in an effort to depoliticize the meeting. "It will guarantee a zoo," one member said. "Like a three-ring circus," said another. The possibility of asking the President to submit a videotaped address to the conference was also received unfavorably. "I think he should either be there, or he shouldn't," was the popular sentiment. Although Dana Van Gorder and Shirley Gross, the Community Task Force's co-chair, argued in favor of the invitation, the scientists were unanimously against it.

Larry Bush, Mayor Art Agnos's right-hand man, spoke up. "You should all realize," he told the scientists on the committee, "that the federal government is the major sponsor of AIDS research, and I would guess that it is the source of most of the grant money for all of you sitting around this table. If you don't invite him, you are sending a message that the scientists want to sit in their ivory tower and not be hassled by the political process.

"You should also be aware," Larry Bush concluded, "that this might be remembered when it comes time for the President to look over AIDS research funding to the NIH."

The effect on the group was stunning. Anyone who thought that scientists don't care about money would have had that impression amended by sitting in that room for ten seconds after Larry Bush's remarks. In an instant, the consensus of the committee changed. "Okay, let's invite him, but make the invitation unattractive so he turns us down," was the resolve of most participants. And so that is what we decided to do. Larry Bush and Shirley Gross volunteered to help me with the letter-writing. Our small group, charged with fashioning an invitation the President *could* refuse, was promptly dubbed the "Just Say No" or the "Thanks But No Thanks" subcommittee.

The Bush issue also came up at a Community Task Force meeting. Shirley Gross reported on the deliberations of the Local Organizing Committee to the group. "We'll be inviting him, but we don't really want him to come," she said, laughing. A number of the other activists, including a few from ACT UP, chimed in. "We don't want him here." There was a lot of bantering back and forth, the activists perversely drafting a hypothetical invitation to Bush that the President would certainly find less than appealing.

Paul Boneberg interjected. "I'm not sure I agree with the whole premise of what you're saying," he told his fellow activists. "I think we want him here. I think we want him here very badly. When the President comes," he continued, "it provides a level of high visibility that will enhance funding opportunities and places AIDS higher on the national agenda. I think we should make every effort to bring him here."

Michelle Roland of ACT UP disagreed. "If he comes, it'll be a big showcase and whitewash. You know very well that if he's here there'll be massive protests and they'll just blame us for them. We shouldn't invite him."

Roland's line of reasoning was intriguing. She was concerned about the negative public image ACT UP would generate if they conducted ugly protests during Bush's visit. Her solution was to discourage Bush's invitation, instead of critically examining whether and how to protest a Presidential visit. Whether she was being doctrinaire (if he comes, we must protest) or was simply recognizing ACT UP's anarchy (even if we wanted to tone down the protests, we can't control our members) was unclear to me.

I listened for a while longer and finally reassured the group that I was writing a letter that would invite the President in a very specific way, making it clear that we wanted him to tackle the tough questions about U.S. AIDS policy for the new decade, including the immigration issue. The Task Force nodded approvingly, but asked to see a copy of the letter. I refused. I could just see this letter being published in the newspaper under a headline saying AIDS CONFERENCE TO IN-VITE PRESIDENT, BUT NOT REALLY. Shirley Gross could be interviewed to describe the "Just Say No" committee that we had jokingly discussed at the organizing group.

In fact, the more I thought about it, the more I realized that I needed to do some political spinning. "I think we should be very clear here," I told the Task Force. "When we do invite the President, it is because we want him to come. The conditions will be very specific, and he may not wish to come under those conditions. But this should not be presented to the press as an invitation designed to have Bush say no."

The invitation letter to the President went through about ten drafts. The final version asked Bush to review the Administration's policies to meet the "scientific, social, and political challenges posed by the AIDS epidemic" in the coming decade. It also mentioned that we were inviting Health and Human Services Secretary Louis Sullivan to address the closing ceremony (thus giving the President his first out) and that, if his schedule did not permit his participation, we would be glad to present a brief videotaped welcoming message (out number two). Although the Vice President was not mentioned by name in the letter, we hoped the between-the-lines message was clear—no Dan Quayle. Read our lips.

All of the staff joined me in saluting and singing "Hail to the Chief" as we dropped the letter into the mailbox. The date was October 26, 1989, only nine days after a devastating earthquake had ravaged San Francisco. If Bush accepted our invitation, I thought as we mailed the letter, we might just be in for another one.

In November 1989, we innocently enjoyed a feeling of control as we awaited the President's reply, not realizing that we sat in the eye of a moving tornado. Relations with the Community Task Force were improving weekly, which allayed our fears of activist disruptions. Larry Kramer's "Uncle Tom" letter would not arrive until a few weeks later; when it did arrive, we found it more amusing than threatening. The October 17th "World Series" earthquake, though disastrous, had claimed fewer lives than originally feared and unleashed a heartwarming response from San Francisco and the nation.

Thankfully, none of our staff was injured, and none of our conference sites or hotels severely damaged.

Most exciting of all, researchers from all over the world sent in their abstracts, and the scientific program began to take shape. It was not until I saw these abstracts that I fully recognized the stunning thematic and geographic breadth of the conference. The first abstract we received was entitled "Tat Protein of Human Immunodeficiency Virus Type I Is Able to Block Tar-mediated Activation of $(2'-5')$ Oligoadenylate Synthetase"; the second was "AIDS: Mass Consciousness and Mass Media in Bulgaria." Eight photocopies of each abstract were requested from authors—an abstract from the Soviet Union came with eight eight-by-ten glossy *photographs* of the paper. More than 4,800 abstracts from about 100 nations followed on the heels of these three papers.

Although most program planning was serious business, there was a lighter side. We received papers enthusiastically touting the healing powers of guided imagery, rectal ozone installation, and the mysterious "Bulgarian Antiviral Substance." A psychologist from Santa Barbara offered to do a presentation on "AIDS and laughter." "If you think your conference may have a tendency to be on the serious side," she wrote, "you might wish to consider a presentation of this sort." Last, I learned that we had competition in the International AIDS Conference business. A group called "Cure AIDS Now" was planning its own conference in Miami Beach to provide an alternative to "the empire builders, grant-grabbers and ego-trippers (better known as the AIDS Mafia)." Their promotion continued: "Cure AIDS Now wishes to invite those who really care to Miami in February 1990 for sun, fun and a gathering of real answers on what must be done."

To our relief, the White House responded to our invitation quickly and negatively. In a letter dated November 14, 1989,

Deputy Assistant for Presidential Appointments Joseph Hagin II passed along the President's regrets "in view of developments in his projected June calendar." June, of course, was more than six months away. Hagin made no mention of the Vice President as a consolation prize. Surprisingly, the request for a videotaped welcome was denied.

With the President on the sidelines, we felt that all our ducks were in a row—our fear of disruption and violence could now be dismissed as paranoia and overreaction. But the feeling was short-lived. Months later, it would be said that George Bush was the first person to boycott the Sixth International Conference on AIDS. In the weeks to come, we learned that he would not be the last.

8 THE BOYCOTT

Since our initial schooling with Hans Paul Verhoef's detention in Minneapolis on April 2, 1989, we had learned much about the politics of AIDS. After having ignored the Verhoef story for nearly a week after it broke, we now realized the importance of paying attention when any news story referred to the conference. So we took quick notice when, on November 23, 1989—Thanksgiving Day—the International Red Cross announced its intention to boycott the San Francisco conference.

From our Americocentric perspective, the INS waiver procedures for HIV-infected travelers—announced in May 1989 just before the Montreal conference—had answered most of the objections to the travel policy. The attention of U.S. scientists and activists quickly turned back to other issues, especially those involving testing and clinical trials of new anti-AIDS drugs. The immigration issue, it seemed, was yesterday's news.

In Europe, however, the passion never died. Representatives of community-based AIDS organizations remained livid over the Byzantine waiver procedure imposed by the U.S. Immigration and Naturalization Service. Their misgivings were legitimate. Anyone wishing to enter the U.S. had to complete a form asking if they had HIV or any other "dangerous and contagious" disease. If they stated that they were HIV-positive and requested a waiver, an unclassified cable was sent to the office of the U.S. Attorney General in Washington, giving details of the person's name, HIV sero-status, and request for a waiver. The decision from Washington took about ten days. If a waiver was granted, the person's passport was stamped with the number 212 (d)(3)(a)(6). This number indicated to INS officials that a waiver had been granted for one of the "dangerous and contagious diseases." In theory this could mean a number of conditions, but in practice it always meant HIV, since anyone with a treatable infectious disease like syphilis or tuberculosis would be encouraged to return after seeking treatment. Not only was the scarlet letter of a person's HIV positivity permanently marked in his or her passport, but it was also recorded in U.S. Embassy records in his or her home country.

The International League of Red Cross Societies, an umbrella organization linking 149 national Red Cross organizations around the world, was the first to boycott. The League acknowledged the importance of the conference and the recent improvements to the U.S. travel policy, but Paer Stenbaeck, secretary-general of the League, said that the revised policy continued to conflict with Red Cross "principles of humanitarian support" for AIDS patients. Participation in the conference, Stenbaeck said, could be construed as condoning discrimination.

Within a week, a number of smaller European community-based organizations, including the World Hemophilia Association, joined the boycott. Sue Lucas, Director of the United Kingdom's Nongovernmental Organization AIDS Consortium, summed up sponsors' concerns. "By offering sponsorship," Lucas wrote to International AIDS Society President Lars Olof Kallings, "the agency may be putting an individual into the position of either identifying him or herself as HIV-positive or breaking the law."

The intensity of feeling in Europe was captured by an editorial in *Lancet*, the popular British medical journal. "The U.S. government has produced a Berlin Wall made of straw and knocked holes in it," the editorial said, referring to the visa waivers. "It is remarkable mainly for its purposelessness and its ugliness. In the middle of next year an international spotlight will be turned on this straw wall when San Francisco hosts the Sixth International Conference on AIDS." Noting the withdrawal by the International Red Cross and World Hemophilia Association, the editorial continued, "It will be interesting to see if other bodies, especially WHO, which has been the international leader in fighting for voluntary confidential testing, have the integrity to protest in the same way."

Although we certainly preferred that the Red Cross and the other European groups be at the conference, those groups' absence by itself could not derail the meeting. Our concern, however, was that the boycott might prove contagious. Just as we had worried six months earlier that a decision by San Francisco's Department of Public Health to withdraw conference sponsorship might steamroll into a political movement, the action by the Red Cross and the other Europeans resurrected the same anxieties—on a global scale. Once again, it was time to network with our allies and hone our sound bites to prevent the boycott from gathering momentum. Our lumbering political machine needed to get back into business.

Dana and I prepared press statements in case the boycott caught fire, but decided not to be too proactive. The meeting was still seven months away. Maybe the press would forget about the immigration issue after a couple of days, and allow us to go back to the conference-planning business. In case the outcry continued, however, we readied our old arguments for the press: The problem is in Washington and not San

Francisco; the conference is critically important; we agree that the policy is wrong and are working to change it; the show must go on. Reporters nearly begged us to get into a shouting match with the Red Cross and other boycotters, but we steadfastly refused to do so. A confrontation might sell newspapers, but it would also intensify the boycott.

It was tempting to be angry at the boycotters. We shared the same frustration as Idaho potato farmers who asked "Why us?" when pro-choice advocates threatened to boycott their spuds over abortion restrictions in their state. "Don't you think boycotting us is inappropriate," conference chair John Ziegler asked me one day, "since we're not an arm of the federal government?"

"This is politics," I answered. "The fifteen hundred members of the press who will be at the meeting make us a strategically appropriate venue for anybody wanting to change *anything* in AIDS." By capturing the attention of the world press, I continued, the boycotters could embarrass the federal government into resurrecting policy discussions on an issue that it hoped it had already laid to rest.

As the *Lancet* editorial had implied, the big unknown in the boycott equation was the World Health Organization. The withdrawal of the Red Cross (which, like the WHO, is based in Geneva) put enormous pressure on the WHO to do the same. From where we sat, the loss of the WHO would be a critical blow, sending a signal to the world that the conference was expendable. I doubted that Jonathan Mann or WHO Director-General Hiroshi Nakajima would wish to send such a signal or to embarrass the U.S. government, since about 20 percent of the organization's budget came from U.S. government contributions. However, the WHO (like its parent, the United Nations) exists at the fickle whim of international politics. If the pressure in Europe mounted, WHO support for the conference could simply evaporate.

A few weeks after the Red Cross announcement, Jonathan Mann's WHO assistant Kathleen Kay came to San Francisco.

She brought with her a statement on HIV travel by WHO's Management Committee, the group's main policy-setting body. The statement was classic WHO-speak. It urged countries to "comply with resolution WHO 41.24 on the need to avoid discriminatory action against and stigmatization of HIV-infected persons and persons with AIDS in the provision of services, employment, and travel." Furthermore, it called on Mann to continue his efforts to change HIV-travel policy (without mentioning the U.S. specifically) and declared that the WHO would review its position on cosponsorship of "international conferences" (without mentioning our conference by name) at its regular April 1990 meeting.

For now, it seemed, the WHO would continue its quiet diplomacy, taking a wait-and-see attitude. Press inquiries to the WHO about the organization's position on the San Francisco conference were met with obfuscation: "We hope there will be a change in the policy." It was particularly important, Kathleen Kay said, to use the correct buzzwords for the press. She briefed us on the WHO's lexicon of no-no's. "We should never say 'boycott' because that tends to generate a momentum of its own," she said. "You should always be talking about groups 'withdrawing their participation' from the conference." Similarly, she instructed us not to talk about the "immigration issue," but to talk simply about the "travel issue." "Immigration implies that you favor people being allowed to become permanent residents in the United States—that's an issue I don't think you want to touch." We agreed. There would be no more attempts to fix the "immigration issue" to end the "boycott"; instead, our crusade was now to fix the "travel issue" to stem the "withdrawal of participation." It seemed that ACT UP was not the only group with its own word police.

In our renewed fight to fix the travel issue, we needed strong allies. We looked to the U.S. National Commission on AIDS for support.

The National Commission had a checkered past. The original commission had been born—stillborn, as it turned out —in 1987 as the Presidential Commission, in response to growing criticism that Ronald Reagan had ignored the epidemic—one that had killed more than twenty thousand Americans before the President mentioned the word "AIDS" in a speech. In 1986, the prestigious Institute of Medicine had recommended that a national AIDS commission be convened to monitor research, health care, public health, legal, and ethical aspects of the epidemic; advise Congress and the President about these issues; and report to the public. The Reagan Administration reluctantly agreed, but began to lower expectations even before the group was constituted. "It would be wrong if anyone thought this body was going to coordinate national AIDS policy," said archconservative Gary Bauer, Reagan's assistant for domestic policy. Bauer was right: The group disbanded soon after its first meeting amid storms of protest over alleged bias against gays and minorities by some of its members.

Retired Navy Admiral James Watkins took over as chair of the Second Presidential Commission. Watkins was promptly labeled by AIDS advocates as an Administration lackey, a conservative who was more likely to moralize than criticize the government. However, Watkins was a military man who insisted on getting things done. His report on the epidemic, released in June 1988, called for nothing less than a revamping of the nation's health care delivery system. The commission, Watkins said, found problems with "many issues— discrimination, nursing shortages, therapeutic drug development, intravenous drug abuse, education—issues that could not be resolved by any short-term solutions. To neglect these would build up long-term health problems that will be much more expensive to resolve in the long run." Watkins's report, though well-received in the AIDS community, was largely ignored by the Reagan Administration, which thanked the admiral for his good work and promptly disbanded the commission. Months later, Watkins was named U.S. Secretary of

Energy, thus ending his fleeting career as an AIDS advocate.

It was a sign of how things had changed in the AIDS world that, in 1989, when the National Commission on AIDS was constituted by Congress to replace the Presidential Commission, June Osborn, a liberal public health expert, could be selected as its chairwoman. Osborn had impeccable credentials. A physician with a background in basic virology, she had moved into the fields of epidemiology and public health years before the first cases of AIDS were reported, rising to become Dean of the highly regarded University of Michigan School of Public Health. She was articulate and spunky—the rare individual praised by both AIDS scientists and activists. She had no shortage of opinions about AIDS discrimination, funding, and prevention, and had the courage to speak her mind. In short, she was perfect for the job, which is why it surprised so many that she got it.

Before the Montreal conference, I called Osborn to solicit her help on the travel issue. "I'd love to help," she said, "but my nomination is up before the Congress now. I can't be too visible. Yet." She promised to work behind the scenes, and she did. By December 1989, her nomination was approved, and she was Chair of the new National Commission on AIDS. Now she could take her gloves off and fight.

Osborn held a press conference on December 12, 1989. U.S. restrictions on travel by HIV-infected people, she said, were "counterproductive, discriminatory, and a waste of resources. They fly in the face of strong international opinion and practice, they lead to unconscionable infringement of human rights and dignity, and they reinforce a false impression that AIDS and HIV infection are a general threat when in fact they are sharply restricted in their mode of transmission." Osborn was joined at the press conference by representatives of the AIDS Action Council, the International Red Cross, and the American Bar Association, all of whom echoed the commission's call for the U.S. to end travel restrictions. The restrictions demanded immediate attention, Osborn said, because they threatened the Sixth International Conference on AIDS.

The press turned its attention to Dana, who attended the Washington, D.C., press conference. How many people might not come to the conference because of the boycott? they asked. "We expected twelve thousand registrants, but we may lose three thousand unless the travel policy is changed," he said. In the weeks that followed, in newspapers ranging from the *San Francisco Chronicle* to the *Wall Street Journal*, the number showed up time and time again, appearing as "three thousand of the possible twelve thousand," in some papers and "one quarter of the anticipated registrants" in others.

I found it amusing, and a bit disconcerting, that the aura of authenticity was granted such a number once it appeared in print. Before Dana left for Washington, he and I had discussed the impact of the boycott. We quickly realized that we had absolutely no idea how many people might participate in the boycott, but guessed it would be more than a thousand and less than five thousand. We settled on the number three thousand as a compromise: high enough (we hoped) to scare the Administration and Congress into fearing that the boycott would capture world attention, while not so high as to panic University of California administrators (whose continued support and funding were critical) into thinking that the meeting was in grave danger of collapsing. Despite the number's genesis from thin air, the press embraced it without challenge. And after enough repetition in print, everyone forgot where they first heard it—fabrication transformed into fact.

With the help of the "three thousand boycotters," the Osborn press conference started the ball rolling anew. All eyes turned back toward Washington for a solution, and once again, denial reigned. The Public Health Service said the ball was in the Justice Department's court, Justice dribbled it to the White House, and the White House bounce-passed it to the Congress. As opposition grew, it became clear that the Administration's balancing act—the attempt to pacify the

AIDS community with the waiver policy without raising the ire of the conservatives—had not worked. More, probably much more, would have to be done if the White House was to avoid a public relations fiasco.

Our hopes that the boycott—er, withdrawal—flap would be limited to Europe were dashed in early December, when the prestigious U.S. National Association of People With AIDS (NAPWA) joined the Europeans. In its press release, NAPWA called on "friends, organizations, scientists, and the medical community to join us in solidarity by withdrawing their participation in the conference; for there can be no substantive conference on AIDS without the participation and consideration of those directly affected by the disease."

The heat was turned up another few degrees with a December *New York Times* op-ed piece by Australian political scientist Dennis Altman and Canadian researcher Andrew Orkin. They described an incident at the border of Vermont and Canada, in which a member of a group carried AIDS literature. "This was taken as suggesting that he was infected with HIV," the authors said, "and therefore not to be admitted to the United States. The party was finally admitted after it became clear that officials did not know how to determine HIV antibody status on sight." The article went on to criticize the U.S., described as the world's largest net exporter of HIV infection, for its exclusionary and discriminatory immigration policy. Congress was stampeded into the ineffective policy, the authors claimed, to show evidence of its "tough-mindedness and control."

The op-ed piece concluded: "The U.S. policy, if unchanged, will pose a dilemma for foreigners who would like to attend the Sixth International Conference on AIDS in San Francisco next June. San Francisco has been an important model in how to respond to the epidemic, and the conference is being organized by some of the world's most respected AIDS experts. Yet many people will not be willing to seek the waivers required by U.S. law for them to attend. And why should they? Accepting a waiver amounts to an implicit acceptance of the discriminatory practice."

As groups like NAPWA and San Francisco's Shanti Project announced their withdrawal from the conference, there was one group that made it clear that they would stick with us like glue. At every turn, ACT UP New York reassured us that they were on board, come hell or high water. The conference, they told us, was simply too valuable to miss.

Like Alice in Wonderland, I struggled to make sense of the topsy-turvy events. In Montreal, it was the scientists who threatened to shun future conferences because of the level of activism and PWA involvement. Now, scarcely six months later, the PWA groups were pulling out; there was even talk of an alternative international PWA/activist conference in Madrid. Ironically, this was precisely what the activists had initially wanted to avoid, since they suspected (correctly, I think) that the level of press coverage for a separate activist conference would be a tiny fraction of that expected in San Francisco. Protesting against the government and the scientists without either group present was akin to one-handed clapping—much activity but little noise.

For the scientists' part, quite a few were elated at the prospect of fewer HIV-infected people and their advocates attending the Sixth International Conference, although none came out and said so publicly. Perhaps the conference (and, by inference, the epidemic) would be returned to its rightful owners, many thought.

By this time, I had become a convert, and was looking forward to the breadth and humanity that a strong PWA presence would bring to the conference. The gathering would be diminished, I thought, by the absence of groups like NAPWA and the Shanti Project, whose volunteers enhanced the quality of life of thousands of AIDS patients.

Although my thinking had evolved, my primary mission was to protect the conference's interests. If ACT UP decided to skip San Francisco in June, *that* was a disappointment I could get over. But in this, the Alice in Wonderland world of AIDS, it was the Shantis and NAPWAs that were heading elsewhere.

With the spread of the boycott to American soil, the Bush Administration recognized the need for quick action. A wild-fire of controversy was burning, and a working group composed of officials from the Departments of Health and Human Services, State, and Immigration convened to douse it. The group's proposed solution in January 1990, unfortunately, was guaranteed to stoke the fire.

For the most part, the working group's fix would have passed a word-police checkpoint, as it had all the politically correct phraseology: It addressed "international concerns about confidentiality," it strived to "avoid documentation that might stigmatize travelers," and it called for "expeditious handling of applications." What was troubling was the group's ultimate goal: "to work within the current legal framework to facilitate *attendance* by HIV-infected persons *at international conferences*" (emphasis added).

The Administration, it appeared, was once again under-estimating the international passion against the travel policy. The working group was correct in thinking that the original objections had been based on the inability of non-American HIV-infected people to participate in our conference. But over time, the issue had become much more than that—it had become a litmus test of the Bush Administration's commit-ment to fighting AIDS discrimination. The time when the problem could be solved by simply finding a way to allow a few hundred PWAs to attend the conference without hassle had long passed. Another quick fix designed to accommodate conference-goers while leaving those travelling to the United States for other reasons exposed to the vagaries of the waiver process could make things even worse than they already were. "A sellout!" people would say. "The government is trying to pacify the organizers and the registrants!" others would cry. And, of course, they would be right. The boycott would continue unabated.

I quickly called Jim Allen, Director of the National AIDS Program Office and the highest ranking AIDS official in the Public Health Service, to let him know what a mistake the Administration would be making if the fix covered only conference delegates. Someone had their signals crossed, Allen said, since the changes he knew to be in the works applied to all HIV-infected travelers. Allen was exasperated by the pressure that he and his office were feeling on the travel issue. "Why doesn't anybody turn to Congress?" he said. "They caused this mess. Why do we have to fix it?"

Allen suggested that we continue to lobby Congress on the issue, concentrating not just on Ted Kennedy, for whom lobbying on HIV travel was singing to the choir, but on swaying Republican Senators Simpson and Hatch. He also recommended that we emphasize the possible cancellation of the smaller World Hemophilia Conference scheduled to take place in Washington in August. His reasons were threefold. First, the World Hemophilia Federation, unlike the San Francisco organizing group, would not go out of business after its conference ended. We might be strong sprinters, but they had the staying power to complete what might turn out to be a marathon race. Second, the hemophilia group had active chapters in every state; if they got their act together, they could produce an effective nationwide blitz to change the policy. Finally, perhaps most important, the hemophilia group was not associated with a gay activist element, an element that could be costing us mainstream support in Washington.

Allen then outlined the predicted changes in the policy. First, when an HIV-infected foreign national applied for a visa, he would continue to have to apply for a waiver. Once he indicated that he had a "dangerous and contagious" disease, however, his application would automatically be handled by a United States foreign officer, not a national of the host country. This would provide, according to Allen, "a degree of confidentiality," since the HIV-infected person would not have to declare his sero-positivity to a foreign national official. Second, the new visa application process would leave no permanent record in the passport—the visa would be torn off so that it and its waiver stamp did not remain as a permanent record of HIV positivity. Finally, the waiver process would be expedited, with foreign officials of the Justice Department authorized to approve applications. Until now, each application had to be routed back through the Department of Justice in Washington, causing a long delay.

I told Allen that these changes, although positive, would not be enough to satisfy the boycotting groups. This would be especially so if they applied only to conference participants and not across the board. The quick fix simply would not do.

With the mixed signals coming out of Washington, one of our most hopeful fronts was Atlanta, where the Centers for Disease Control debated a proposal to remove all diseases except active tuberculosis from the list of "dangerous and contagious diseases." After all, said some CDC staffers, tuberculosis was the only disease on the list that truly was dangerous and contagious—that is, it could be caught via casual contact from a cough. One had to engage in volitional high-risk activities like unsafe sexual intercourse and sharing infected needles to contract all of the other diseases on the list, including HIV. Our sources at the CDC told us that Assistant Health Secretary and former CDC top gun James Mason supported the plan to revise the list and was trying to muster political backing before going public with it. The CDC could, by itself, drop the sexually transmitted diseases like gonorrhea and syphilis from the list. But HIV infection, added by Congressional statute, could not be deleted without another act of Congress. At least, so claimed the Administration.

No one was particularly hopeful that Congress could gather the momentum to change the law in time for the conference. After all, the Helms amendment had passed 97 to 0. Even if the Senators had believed they were voting on HIV immigration and not travel, it was going to take a massive lobbying effort to win a new vote. Time was running short.

Our best hope rode on the shoulders of Michael Iskowitz, Senator Ted Kennedy's talented staffer on the Committee on Labor and Human Relations. It is axiomatic in Washington that all important Congressional action is generated by staff men and women working behind the scenes, attending to the details of legislation. Hedrick Smith, in his classic book *The Power Game*, described the role of the staffer: "Many people, not understanding how the game is played, are dazzled by political celebrities and feel they have to go to the top: to the president or his right-hand man, to the Treasury secretary, the senator, the committee chairmen. . . . The insiders pay their respects to the person with the title and then work the serious issues with less-celebrated staff people who actually draft policy."

We went to Iskowitz to try to move things along in the Senate. Perhaps Senator Kennedy could hold Senate hearings on the HIV-travel restrictions, and ask Mason and officials from the CDC to testify about the wrongheadedness of the current policy. At first, we were encouraged. But as time passed and we saw little movement, we realized that each of our potential allies, such as Kennedy in the Senate and Henry Waxman and Barney Frank in the House, was gingerly ushering his own pet bill through the dance of legislation. None, it seemed, including Iskowitz, wanted to risk the wrath of Senator Helms and the other conservatives over the HIV-travel issue. Helm's power to be prickly—his porcupine power—was once again winning the day.

Just as Helms passed the travel restrictions in 1987 by

attaching them to a popular bill, we searched for a bill on the Congressional fast track on which to hitch a revision of the CDC list. In one half-baked scheme, we considered linking a revision of the list to a bill—steamrolling through Congress at the time—that would allow Chinese students displaced by the massacre in Tienanmen Square to remain in America. We became more and more willing to grasp at straws like these as the shadow cast by the boycott grew longer.

The International AIDS Society was a paper tiger. First conceived at the Second International Conference on AIDS in Paris in 1986 and founded two years later, its primary mission was to bless and organize the series of international conferences. But it quickly ran into a classic catch-22—no one was quite certain what the IAS did, and thus no one was willing to give it enough money to allow it to do very much. And so that is exactly what it did—not very much. Its leadership was a who's who of international AIDS researchers and clinicians, and its president, Swede Lars Olof Kallings, a dedicated and charismatic potentate. But Kallings, who with his long face and white goatee looks like Hollywood's idea of the European professor, was a Wizard of Oz, presiding over a land more of illusion than reality.

When the series of international conferences left Paris for Stockholm, Montreal, and San Francisco, the IAS continued in its role as an international cosponsor. But the struggling organization could not give what it did not have. So its contributions were limited to a few thousand dollars and the valuable advice provided by Kallings and Executive Secretary Friedrich Deinhardt of Germany. With its staff of one secretary and tiny budget, it could do little else.

But perception is often more important than reality, and few outside the AIDS inner circle recognized the Lilliputian nature of the IAS. Often, the IAS and the World Health Organization were spoken of in tandem, as if of equal stature —the speaker failing to appreciate the vastness of the Geneva operation, with its billion-dollar budget and thousands of employees. Moreover, smallness has its virtues. The IAS could nimbly convene its board, debate a controversial issue, and draft a resolution in a few weeks' time, while WHO parliamentarians might still be haggling over which committee had jurisdiction.

All of this is to explain how it was that the IAS's deliberations on the boycott held the power to sway world opinion and determine the WHO's position, despite the mismatch in size and stature between the two organizations. The IAS, by meeting early and deciding quickly, was like the Iowa or New Hampshire Presidential primary—its influence far out of proportion to its size.

Paul Volberding, IAS board member and the organization's President-elect, returned from three days of IAS meetings in Berlin in late December. Berlin had the smell of history in the making. Each day brought new reports of staggering political upheaval as the walls of Eastern Europe crashed down. On the day of Volberding's return, the Brandenburg Gate, the site of the last days of the Third Reich, was breached, allowing free passage between East and West Germany. It was ironic, perhaps prophetic, that Berlin in December 1989 was the site of some of the most important discussions regarding the free passage of HIV-infected individuals across national borders.

Volberding sat down with Dana and me to describe the IAS deliberations. He had a pained look on his face. "We have some big trouble here, boys," he said. He described how Kallings and Deinhardt, though strong supporters of the conference, were beginning to sway with the strong breeze in Europe. "They say that unless the U.S. policy changes drastically, they're going to have to pull out of the conference."

"You mean future conferences like Boston's," I half-declared and half-asked, referring to the 1992 conference. It was already widely expected that the IAS and the WHO would withdraw their support for the Boston conference if the restrictions weren't lifted. But Boston was nearly three years away—time enough for Congress to change the law and allow the Eighth International Conference on AIDS to take place on American soil.

"*All* conferences," Volberding said sadly. "They don't feel that they can possibly distinguish between the San Francisco conference and future conferences in the United States. If the policy is wrong, they feel like they may need to drop their support for our meeting. My read from them is that they are not going to budge. These guys are playing hardball."

It was even bleaker than that. Lars Kallings chaired the Global Commission on AIDS, which advises the WHO on policy matters. The WHO Management Committee was planning to evaluate its continued sponsorship of our meeting in April 1990, four months away and a mere two months before the conference. Volberding sketched a nasty picture, in which Kallings and some of the other Europeans forced the hand of the WHO to withdraw its support for *all* conferences in countries that discriminate against HIV-positive individuals. Such a resolution would bind the WHO into withdrawing its support from the San Francisco conference.

Dana, Paul, and I began to play out worst-case scenarios. By this time, we had all taken on pride of ownership for the conference; each of us had a strong interest in seeing our efforts bear fruit. What would happen if the IAS and the WHO both pulled out in April, a prospect that seemed, for the first time, believable? The conversation turned Machiavellian.

"You'd think from sitting here," I said, "that the travel issue was all that anyone was talking about in the world of AIDS. But you know damn well that ninety-eight percent of the scientists and clinicians in the world haven't heard of this debate." I pointed out that we already had nearly a thousand conference registrants, and the abstracts were coming in fast and furious. I continued. "My guess is that by April we'll have judged five thousand abstracts, and about eight thousand registrants will have signed up." At that point, we'd be talking about the meeting as a viable living, breathing organism, not a theoretical possibility. We'd be aware of any major research findings that would not see the light of day in a timely fashion if the conference was cancelled. We might go down, but at least we'd go down fighting—touting the importance of the conference and the tragedy of its passing to the world press.

Looming as ominously as a WHO and IAS withdrawal in April 1990 was the specter that UCSF, our main sponsor, might lose its nerve. So far, the university had remained terrifically supportive despite the political ill winds. But as the sea grew choppier, would this politically conservative institution be able to stand the swell, or would it opt to cut its losses and cast off? It would take tremendous courage on the part of university administrators to continue pouring millions into a conference that had become a pariah in the eyes of the world AIDS community. As we contemplated the worst-case scenario, we knew that it was unrealistic to count on UCSF's continued support if the international cosponsors pulled out.

So in the final analysis, the worst-case scenario seemed likely to translate into the scrapping of the San Francisco conference. Moreover, it seemed possible that it might mean the end of the series of international conferences—a major blow to the global fight against AIDS. It was easy enough to plan to hold conferences in countries that lacked discriminatory laws, but laws change quickly and potential funders might think twice once they recognized that their $3 million up-front investment could become worthless overnight by dint of a boycott over a political issue. And there was no guarantee that HIV-travel restrictions would remain the issue *du jour*. Perhaps next year's issue would be a slow approval process for new drugs, unavailable health insurance, or discrimination in the workplace. Such a fickle political environment provides barren soil for investors.

Now that we had worked ourselves into a lather over the consequences of an IAS/WHO mutiny, we considered the likelihood of such a scenario. It was hard to think of a player in the boycott game who would benefit from the conference's cancellation over the travel issue. The conference represented the only visible product of the IAS, its *raison d'être*. For the WHO, concerned with the global battle to control AIDS as well as with its own internal need to justify its existence and budget, the conference provided a week-long international scrutiny of the ongoing devastation of the epidemic and a showcase for the organization's labor. A global boycott leading to the decimation of the conference would certainly focus the world's spotlight on the travel issue, an important goal. However, without a conference there would be no focal point for the world's press to congregate and reflect on the state of the global battle, and the research and public health agenda on AIDS would be essentially forgotten for the year 1990.

Even the activists, in a perverse way, had a strong incentive to preserve the conference. Because of their successes, the San Francisco conference would be more to their liking than any previous conference, providing tangible evidence of their political clout and, to their minds, the rightness of their cause. More important, it would bring fifteen hundred members of the press into town, a ready spotlight for their protests.

Paul Boneberg sent a letter from our Community Task Force to AIDS advocacy and activist groups all over America in defense of the conference. The letter, which asked the groups not to boycott, spoke of the conference organizers' inclusion of HIV-infected people in planning, our strong commitment to resolving the travel problem, and the importance of the conference to the global fight against AIDS. When I saw Boneberg's letter, I scribbled a note on it for Dana. "I'm sure there is a heavy quid pro quo here," I wrote, "but what the hell. This is better press than I get from my mother." True to form, the quid pro quo came a few days later when Boneberg warned us of the fragility of the activists' support and the possibility of disruptions if we weren't more forthcoming on free passes to the conference for people with AIDS.

"Let me understand you," Dana said to Boneberg. "The conference is very important, and you want to preserve it. However, if you succeed in preserving it, then you may spend most of your time there disrupting it." "Yeah, that's about right," said Boneberg.

The bottom line, then, was that an IAS pullout was possible, it might be a harbinger of a WHO desertion, and the combination would be the conference's death knell. Yet none of it was likely to happen, because it was not in any of the players' interest for it to happen. Dana, Paul, and I congratulated ourselves on our thorough analysis of the situation and breathed a collective sigh of relief. There really was nothing to worry about.

But then why, when we left the room, did we scramble to find the phone number of Lloyd's of London to price cancellation insurance?

If we were concerned about losing the support of the IAS and the WHO, the organizers of the 1992 Boston conference were terrified. Just as the reality of our conference—now a mere six months away, with thousands of registrations and scientific papers already submitted—would in some ways prove to be our salvation, the Harvard University organizers of the 1992 conference feared that the abstractness of their effort would prove their downfall.

The Boston organizers were as naive about the politics of the conference as we had been during our embryonic stage. At the Montreal conference, they had trotted out their promotional material—a glossy poster in which Harvard and its VERITAS shield took top billing over the 1992 conference itself. From the resounding criticism that greeted the poster, they learned that institutional hubris was a fatal flaw when it came to this meeting, and quickly toned down the self-promotion.

The Harvard organization differed from ours, in that most of the ground work was being done by a nonphysician. Alan Fein, an M.B.A. who served as the Executive Director of

Harvard's AIDS Institute, was charged with making the Boston conference a reality. After the foundation was laid, the scientists, led by prominent retrovirologist and conference Chair Max Essex, would step in to plan the science. An earnest and unpretentious man, Fein was very concerned about the boycott and its potential impact on the Boston effort. He was aware that the WHO and the IAS were getting skittish. We spoke one morning in early January 1990.

I told Fein that my assessment of the situation was that the two international cosponsors might decide to continue to support the San Francisco conference but put Boston on the chopping block. "The pressure on them to do something is intense," I said. "If they say that San Francisco is a go, they may need to say that they won't support any *future* conferences in countries with discriminatory travel policies." Furthermore, I told Fein, I didn't see any way that the Boston conference could survive an IAS/WHO pullout.

"Isn't it likely that the academics will come if it's a good conference, even if the PWAs and activists stay away because of the travel issue?" Fein asked.

"Alan, I'm afraid it doesn't work that way," I said, recalling the good old days when I too believed life was so simple. "If the activists are pissed off about HIV travel and don't want Boston to happen, they may not be there . . . but they'll *be there*," I said.

The Boston group was determined to profit from our political experience. One of their first acts after forming their local organizing committee was to invite a few members of the local gay community to serve. It had been a challenge to find gays willing to oblige, Fein told me; many worried openly about being co-opted. "This is going to be tough," he lamented. "Harvard has a terrible relationship with the local community."

But what the Boston group lacked in community relations and AIDS political experience, they made up in Washington connections. San Francisco and Boston both have powerful medical communities, and UCSF and Harvard are each one of the handful of top medical centers in the country. When it came to relative clout in the nation's corridors of power, however, there was no question that Harvard ranked head and shoulders above UCSF and everyone else. Over time, as the Boston crowd became convinced that its conference would be cancelled if the U.S. travel policy wasn't changed, the old boys' network went into action.

Many Washington politicos have, at one time or another, spent time in Cambridge, Massachusetts, often as students at Harvard's Law School or John F. Kennedy School of Government. One such politico was Attorney General Richard Thornburgh, who for months had been ignoring our requests for a meeting. Within days, Harvard President Derek Bok had an audience with Thornburgh to discuss the travel issue. The early attempt by Mike Iskowitz to schedule Senate hearings on the issue had fizzled; the Kennedy staffer no longer returned our frequent calls. But the calls from Boston were quickly returned, and soon Senator Kennedy was pushing harder than ever to change the policy.

For the most part, we worked side-by-side with Fein and the Harvard organizers. Our synergy was impressive, but deceptive. In the back of each of our minds was the strong possibility that the U.S. government, the WHO, and the IAS would choose the expedient route, begrudgingly supporting our conference while jettisoning Harvard's—a powerful lamb sacrificed on the altar of the international politics of AIDS.

While Harvard's involvement raised the heat in Washington, the AIDS community neared its boiling point. As 1990 began, increasingly frustrated community groups demanded action even as reports from Washington continued to suggest that changes were forthcoming. The withdrawal by NAPWA and Shanti had forced many AIDS community-based organizations to put down their nickel—were they for the conference or against it? The San Francisco AIDS Foundation was in; New York's Gay Men's Health Crisis was out. Fence-sitting became more and more untenable, the tone of the debate increasingly strident.

Even our own Community Task Force rebelled. The Task Force's letter to American AIDS groups asking them to delay a boycott decision had not—we learned—been approved by all Task Force members, and many were highly critical of Paul Boneberg for failing to solicit their input. Moreover, even Task Force Cochair Leon McKusick, who had worked closely with us since Montreal, threatened to jump ship.

In a year-end letter to Ziegler and Volberding, McKusick criticized the conference cochairs for refusing to provide twelve hundred free passes to allow HIV-infected people to attend the conference (after vigorous internal debate we had settled on 375, hundreds more than any previous meeting) and for not working hard enough to fix the travel issue. "We are willing to help the 1990 conference shape a response to the boycott," wrote McKusick. "However, our members will only support the goals of individuals whose thoughts and actions basically align with the collective values of the Task Force. We also seek collaboration with individuals who celebrate the participation of those who are HIV-infected. . . . In these matters, the Task Force is not at all clear where you stand." The letter concluded with a pleasant but gratuitous invitation for further discussion.

We were livid. "You just can't win with these guys," Volberding said. "What the hell do they want me to do—go to the Justice Department and get arrested? We've done everything we can."

I agreed. "We ask these people to see all sides of the issue," I said, "but that's just not what they do. They are political animals, and if you give them ninety-nine percent of what they want but hold back on one percent, you'll be hearing about that one percent until they knock down the walls of the conference."

Volberding understood the politics better than almost anyone in America, but continued to seethe. "Look at the Stockholm meeting [the Fourth International Conference on AIDS]," he said. "At Stockholm, all of the PWA issues and all of the social issues were relegated to the 'Face of AIDS' programs, which were sandwiched between the scientific sessions. The activists complained bitterly about it, but what do you hear about the Stockholm meeting? You basically hear that it was a good meeting. Maybe we should remember that as we decide whether we need to make more concessions to the activists."

In early January 1990, news of more community groups withdrawing from the conference dribbled in. But as long as the boycott wasn't tarnishing the program that was beginning to crystallize, we remained sanguine about the prospects for a successful meeting. Abstracts from all over the world continued to pile up in our office, and our invitations to major speakers were generally met with acceptance.

But there were some chinks in the program's armor. We had invited Belinda Mason, the HIV-infected homemaker who served as NAPWA's president and as a member of June Osborn's National AIDS Commission, to speak at a plenary session. Her topic: the perspectives of HIV-infected people related to the development of new AIDS drugs. Predictably, Mason joined NAPWA in withdrawing from the conference, saying that she felt obliged to "join my fellow PWA/HIV-positives around the world in global solidarity. . . ."

A more surprising, and more passionate, letter came from Herbert Daniel, the HIV-infected chairman of pela VIDDA, a support organization for PWAs in Brazil. Daniel thanked us for inviting him to speak at the conference's closing ceremony. "When I found myself face-to-face with AIDS," the activist recalled, "the horror soon gave way to a stronger love of life, and living became infinitely richer. I also discovered that my fight would gain force if shared with others—not only to better live with illness and death, but to better confront the prejudice and the discrimination brought on by the epidemic, often more deadly than the virus itself.

"This passion for living has made me particularly sensitive to the many forms of 'opportunistic discrimination' that resurface with AIDS. . . . The current American visa policy directed at the detection and penalizing of people who are HIV-infected or living with AIDS, alleging the protection of those 'healthy others,' provokes my deepest indignation. Its discriminatory content deepens the chasm between 'us and them' and works against solidarity—the only vaccine we can count on today for AIDS.

"As it stands, I feel that I cannot justly accept the invitation. It would violate my innermost principles, undermine my work, and that of hundreds of groups and nongovernmental organizations who strive to protect the rights and the dignity of all people living with AIDS—with no exceptions. To be an exception, as would be my case at the conference, no matter how personally rewarding, is precisely the crux of the issue at stake. All of humanity has in some way been touched by the infection, and can no longer be impartial to the pain, the desolation, and the isolation caused by the discriminatory measures associated with AIDS."

Our fears of a world-wide boycott movement among community groups were allayed slightly by another letter from Brazil, this one from a group called Grupo de Apoio à Prevenção da AIDS (GAPA). Gerson Barreto Winkler, the group's president, criticized the U.S. travel policy and called for its revision. But, he said, attending the Sixth Conference could serve to "strengthen the international effort against AIDS and deepen the discussions on critical social and public policy issues as well. . . . The withdrawal of community-based AIDS support groups, especially those from developing countries, is a mistaken decision that threatens the power of the conference to enhance the global response to the epidemic."

The debate—to boycott or not to boycott—raged in our own backyard as well as in Brazil. A graphic showing the conference logo (a stylized picture of the AIDS virus) covered by a large question mark accompanied a January article in the San Francisco *Bay Guardian*. "It seems quite possible that U.S. immigration policy could dominate a five-million-dollar conference that was dedicated not only to vital AIDS medical and research discoveries, but community and policy issues as well," said *Guardian* writer David Israels. "That's an eventuality that nobody, not the conference organizers, the boycotters, or even some parts of the U.S. government, really wants—and nobody seems to know how to stop."

But the editorial writer for the *Bay Area Reporter* knew how to stop the eventuality—cancel the boycott. "The Conference is *not* affiliated with our government," said the editorial, "and the conference organizers are diligently working to overcome the many obstacles thrown at them by a careless administration. The organizers are also working to include community-based groups, HIV-infected people, and other groups not usually served by its various programs. Let's give them a chance and not shoot ourselves in the foot once again."

But even as the debate raged within the activist community, acceptances by scientists followed one after another. Sure, rumors about scientific defections were swirling about. According to one, Luc Montagnier would, on his way to the United States for the conference, falsely declare that he was HIV-positive. The resulting international uproar would, it was hypothesized, shame the U.S. government into action.

This rumor was dismissed as completely off the wall until we received a letter from Montagnier in late January. In it, the discoverer of HIV noted "growing concern among European scientists and international organizations about the discriminatory measures taken by U.S. immigration authorities for sero-positive participants. If this problem is not rapidly solved," Montagnier continued, "several international organizations and scientists, including myself, may withdraw their participation."

I had little doubt that Montagnier would decide to come,

as he eventually did. But in January 1990, as we awaited the coming changes in the travel policy, his hesitation was our trump card, to be used if we needed to increase the growing pressure on Washington. For the time being, we kept the Luc card hidden, since widespread knowledge that the French scientist was wavering might backfire on us and cause other scientists to withdraw—not because of objections to the travel issue but because of a perception that the meeting might not be scientifically worthwhile.

Whereas on Wall Street, the passing of inside information is an indictable offense, in Washington it simply represents the nation's capital at work. So mused Hedrick Smith in *The Power Game.* News leaks are a Washington staple—the *New York Times* and *Washington Post* often serve as ersatz message boards upon which the government posts its business for outside review. "Those who are in control of policy," wrote Smith, a *Times* reporter and thus the repository and distributor of scores of leaks, ". . . will try desperately to keep the information loop small, no matter what the issue; those who are on the losing side internally will try to widen the circle."

Once the changes in the HIV-travel policy were announced, it was clear that those in Washington pushing for substantive change were the losers. Their attempt to widen the circle of information surfaced on the pages of the *New York Times* on January 17, 1990. As Jim Allen had predicted, the changes reported in the *Times* leak provided for increased confidentiality for HIV-infected individuals declaring their seropositivity, an expedited waiver process, and the stamping of a separate document (not the passport) indicating that the bearer was HIV-infected.

But closer scrutiny of the changes revealed that they were yet another patch on a tattered shirt of a policy. The shunting of foreign nationals declaring their HIV positivity away from local officials and to American officials was advertised as a step forward, but many questioned whether it really would ensure confidentiality. Similarly, many wondered whether names entered into the INS database might still be accessible to foreign officials. The waivers would be valid for only thirty days; that had not changed. The INS declared proudly that passports would not be stamped, but this would be so only if travelers specifically asked for them not to be stamped. Finally, as we feared, these small changes would apply only to individuals traveling to the Sixth International Conference on AIDS and the World Hemophilia Federation confab.

AIDS organizations and leaders were quick to criticize the Administration. "They have taken the path of least resistance by not going further," said Jean McGuire of the AIDS Action Council, "and that may just excite a louder call for change. It is a real disappointment." Representative Henry Waxman called the changes "well-intentioned, but still discriminatory. I don't know why the Administration doesn't just admit that the World Health Organization, the International Red Cross, and the National Commission are right," he said.

Duke Austin, spokesman for the INS, responded. "I don't see any evidence that the American public is embarrassed whatsoever, outside of these activists," Austin said. "We've had a list of contagious diseases to screen for since back before the turn of the century. Diseases that are not as onerous or dangerous as the AIDS virus—leprosy and syphilis for example. To maintain that list but remove AIDS seems contradictory since AIDS can kill you. Besides, we are very generous in granting the waivers." The U.S. Public Health Service seemed to agree. "The INS deserves bouquets, not brickbats, for these changes," said PHS spokesman Jim Brown. "They have gone as far as they can under current law. It's up to Congress to change the law."

The Administration had, once again, opted for an incremental change, a trial balloon. With the leak to the *Times*, someone was testing the political waters. The hue and cry, at least initially, appeared manageable. So the Bush Administration declared that it had done all it could; further action would have to come from Congress. If the tune sounded familiar, it was. But for the time being, the audience hummed along, turning desperately to the legislators to transpose the notes in a way that might save the San Francisco conference.

No one expected the boycott to die with the INS changes, and it did not. Disappointed, we and the Boston organizers called Iskowitz again, encouraging him to push Kennedy's Senate hearings forward. In anticipation of the hearings, Iskowitz met with high-level staffers from the offices of Senators Hatch and Simpson. The meeting was a disaster. According to reliable sources, the Republican staffers were vehemently opposed to loosening the restrictions on HIV travel. "Why should we let them in here just so they can come and wreak havoc?" said one of the staffers.

INS officials present at the meeting were emboldened to hold their ground, since further change, it appeared, would not be forced upon them by Congress. Kennedy cancelled his hearings, fearing that comments like those made by the Simpson and Hatch staff members might lead to a *tightening* of the travel restrictions. Washington lobbyists approached gay Representative Barney Frank to bring the issue up in the House, where they expected greater support than the Senate. But Frank, distracted by a House Ethics Committee inquiry and preferring not to divert attention from another immigration bill he was sponsoring, declined.

With the Administration again finger-pointing in the direction of Capitol Hill, and Congressional momentum stalled, it appeared that we had reached a dead end. At least we had survived past January 22nd, the last day for abstract submission, and we now had nearly five thousand high-quality abstracts and a similar number of registrants on board. It was time to throw in the towel. We had done all we could with the travel issue, and we now needed to focus attention on the importance of the conference program to the fight against AIDS. Like a bloodied and exhausted boxer, we were incapable of further offense. All our energy would be concentrated on holding on to the ropes and not falling down.

Europe, we knew, would not be as willing to passively take the punches. We waited for the Europeans to emerge from their corner swinging, and soon they did.

We were terribly concerned about what the IAS and the WHO might do in response to the anemic travel-policies changes. The international politics of AIDS was at stake, and the two groups were the major players in that arena.

But there was a bigger arena that we had ignored—the one involving flags, diplomats, and departments of state. In late January, the battle over HIV-travel restrictions reached the governments of the nation-states of Europe. The first salvo came from an unlikely source.

The European Parliament has been called a debating club. Others have slyly observed that what the Parliament does best is lunch. Even its own President, Enrique Barón Crespo, mocked it as "a marginal institution able only to speak but not to make decisions."

The impotence of the Parliament is in part due to logistical inefficiency: Its operations are divided between Brussels, Luxembourg, and Strasbourg. To conduct its monthly meetings in Strasbourg, hundreds of boxes of documents must be sent from Brussels and hundreds of bureaucrats from Luxembourg, at an annual cost of $65 million. Once the meetings begin, the chaos only grows as the Parliament spews out resolutions in a mind-boggling nine official languages. "At the moment, we're on the verge of collapse," Mr. Barón told the *New York Times* in early 1990. "We have to squeeze forty-five agenda items into one week. Sometimes I have to limit speakers to ninety seconds each."

The European Parliament's problems, however, are larger than geography. Members lament their lack of legal authority to shape legislation and influence events, especially at a time when European politics is undergoing such cataclysmic changes as the democratization of Eastern Europe and the 1992 creation of a common European market.

The changes have provided new momentum for the Parliament, and some have begun to speak of its nascent power —the power to be a governing body for a united Europe. With the June 1989 election of a number of well-known politicians—including former French President Valéry Giscard d'Estaing and five former European Prime Ministers— the Parliament's political influence had grown. Amidst the deprecatory remarks about the Parliament, there was a sense of growing respect, if not for its authority then at least for its potential.

On January 18, 1990, one day after the leak of the new waiver policy appeared in the *New York Times*, the European Parliament took up the matter of the U.S. policy on HIV travel. The resolution that resulted was unambiguous. The Parliament, said the resolution, "calls on the U.S. Government to abolish this discriminatory measure concerning access to its territory; calls on all scientists in the European Community not to participate in this conference; calls on nongovernmental and governmental organizations in the Community to do the same; and proposes that the organizers transfer the conference to a country where such discrimination would not take place."

The action by the Parliament caused the U.S. State Department, for the first time, to take notice of a diplomatic brushfire that could rapidly turn into a conflagration. A few days later, a cable was sent from the American Embassy in Paris to the Secretary of State, Washington, D.C. In it, U.S. Ambassador to France Walter Curley informed Secretary James Baker of the decision by the European Parliament. Ominously, he noted that the French Health Minister, Claude Evin, "will not attend the San Francisco International Conference on AIDS unless U.S. visa policies concerning HIV-seropositive individuals and persons with AIDS are changed."

The cable quoted an interview Evin gave to the French daily paper, *Libération*. "It's a question of principle," said the Health Minister. "Tolerance is essential to prevent exclusionary attitudes that no epidemiological or scientific argument justify. I know the importance of holding this conference in San Francisco, but I cannot go there if nothing changes." The cable ended with a section entitled "Comment": "It is not clear whether the modifications in visa procedures that are reportedly under consideration will be sufficient to make the French change their minds about a boycott," wrote Ambassador Curley.

A January 22 State Department cable sent to diplomatic posts around the world described the changes in visa procedures; they were identical to those reported in the *Times* five days earlier. The State Department, said the cable, "does not expect these changes to satisfy everyone who objects to the U.S. Government restrictions on admissions of persons with HIV/AIDS. However, we believe that this is as much as we can do within the limits of the law as it now stands." The name typed at the bottom of the cable was "Baker."

We watched in despair as the nations of Europe withdrew in lockstep (Switzerland withdrew soon after France), and awaited the IAS's response to the visa changes. On February 1, 1990, IAS President Kallings called for an extraordinary meeting of the Advisory Board in Geneva on March 9. "The IAS has now reached a crossroad in its work," Kallings wrote gravely. "It has come to a juncture at which important decisions must be made with regard to its role, contribution, and responsibility."

It was easy to get caught up in all the activity swirling around the travel issue. Each day, it seemed, brought fresh news: another group joining the boycott, a clarification from the U.S. government, a comment from a scientist. I was frustrated, not so much by the situation itself and its impact on the conference as by a nagging sense that there was a cause or connection that we simply didn't understand.

How odious, really, was the travel policy? Of course it was not justified by medical facts, and it could result in the loss of dignity and confidentiality for people travelling to the U.S. On the other hand, the changes announced by the U.S. State Department, though puny, still guaranteed that most HIV-infected people who wished to attend our conference would be able to do so without undue hassle. There were so many other shocking examples of injustice and discrimination—so many other issues that might benefit from the outrage of the world's AIDS and diplomatic communities. In the U.S., for instance, HIV-infected people were subjected to discrimination over jobs, housing, and insurance. Where was the outrage? Why this issue? And why now?

Europe. Somehow, the missing piece of the puzzle involved Europe, and its relationship with America. Finally, the connection dawned on me. This was not so much about facilitating travel by HIV-infected people, or even about discrimination against PWAs, I realized. Before AIDS, there was no love lost between Europe and the U.S.—especially France and the U.S.—but the tension generally lay hidden beneath the surface. In AIDS, however, a field in which the French resent the U.S. government and research community for having—so they believe—purloined credit for the discovery of the causative virus, the wound was raw and the bitterness undisguised. Against the backdrop of the Gallo-Montagnier fracas, it seemed the French (whether consciously or not) were waiting to pick a fight with the United States. What could be better than this pretext—a discriminatory travel policy that threatened the free flow of medical and scientific information? A diplomatic hanging curve ball. Europe, and especially the French, seized the opportunity to wrap themselves in the flag of righteousness and elevate the travel restriction issue to a test of moral integrity.

This insight also dawned on Paul Volberding, especially after he received the letter indicating that the IAS might withdraw from the conference. Paul was acutely aware that there were more important issues to confront in the world of AIDS than travel. He began to feel that on this issue, the IAS was not representing the world AIDS community but simply the European AIDS community. With each passing day, he became more and more galled by the possibility of IAS's withdrawal from the conference, and finally he made up his mind. "I will resign as President-elect if the group votes to boycott," he told me in early February.

The consequences of an IAS withdrawal and a Volberding resignation were frightening. Almost without question, IAS would divide into two—a European AIDS society and an American AIDS society. Where the rest of the world would align itself was anyone's guess, but it almost did not matter. The global fight against AIDS would be irreparably harmed.

The relationship between the scientists and activists, I now realized, was not the only fragile coalition we were fighting to preserve. The events of the coming months could drive a wedge between the European and American AIDS communities. Only further movement from Washington could bridge the widening rift.

In the pre-boycott days, when we asked the organizers of the Stockholm and Montreal conferences what their biggest headache was, they always had one answer: international travel. By this they meant the organizational nightmare of making travel arrangements to bring hundreds of speakers to the conference from faraway places like Malaysia and Zimbabwe. They strongly suggested that we convene a meeting of the organizations that had agreed to sponsor international travelers to the conference—the WHO, the IAS, the United States Agency for International Development (USAID), the Pan-American Health Organization (PAHO) and the Fogarty Center of the NIH. At this meeting, each group could share its insights and begin the knotty process of brokering individual speakers who might be eligible for dual sponsorship.

Jeff Harris and Linda Valleroy, who run the AIDS program

for USAID, were kind enough to sponsor such a meeting in Washington, D.C., on February 22, 1990. When the meeting was originally scheduled months earlier, we had obsessed over the scope of sponsored travel. By February, however, the logistics of distributing per diem checks and facilitating airport connections seemed downright serene compared to the growing panic over HIV travel.

Part of the meeting did serve its original intent, and was quite constructive. All of the sponsors agreed to share lists of travelers and work together to expedite arrangements. We also resolved to develop a plan for a contingency described by Lydia Bond of PAHO. Bond recalled a group of ten Iraqis who simply showed up at the Montreal conference asking for sponsorship. "I ended up paying for them with my Visa card," sighed Bond.

But the issues on everyone's mind were the HIV-travel restrictions and the growing boycott. Dr. Peter West of the State Department and Clyde Howard of the INS were the lions sent by their agencies for sacrifice—they were charged with explaining the Administration's position to a room full of angry international AIDS leaders.

After recounting the histories of the dangerous and contagious disease list, the Helms amendment, and the Verhoef case, West described the interagency working group (which included representatives of the Departments of State, Health, and Justice) that had developed the January changes to the travel policy.

Was there any opportunity to do more within the existing law? West was asked. Yes and no, he answered. He described the bureaucratic obstacle course that would have to be negotiated before further action was possible. The Department of State, under intense diplomatic pressure after the European Parliament and French government withdrawals, had recently asked the Public Health Service to state its position on whether HIV-infected travelers posed a significant health risk to the U.S. public. If PHS said they did not, explained West, and this passed muster within the State Department, then it would be up to the Department of Justice to approve the legal arrangements. If Justice deemed it legal to remove HIV from the dangerous and contagious list, then the political aspects of the decision, which would almost certainly be adjudicated at 1600 Pennsylvania Avenue, would be decisive.

We asked about the possibility of a legislative change. West felt that this was unlikely to take place before our conference, but stood a good chance afterward, since both the CDC and Assistant Health Secretary James Mason were now known to favor converting the entire list of dangerous and contagious diseases to one containing "conditions of public health significance" that would, for now, include only one disease: active tuberculosis. Although the CDC recommended the removal of AIDS, but not HIV, from the list, its real position was clear but stated only off the record: The agency would also remove HIV from the list had it the authority to do so.

Soon the discussion became more politically charged. Glen Margo of AIDSCOM said that the reactions to the travel policy seen up to this point were "small waves in a tidal pool, but this is going to turn into a tsunami." Lars Kallings spoke of the boycott becoming a "chain reaction." "This could be the end of international conferences," the IAS president said. "The atmosphere in Europe is very different. People are making snap decisions." The INS's computer list, which contained the names of all individuals granted an HIV waiver, was described by William Haseltine of Harvard as "apartheid in the United States." West and Howard listened to the criticism and promised to take it back to the interagency working group. But neither held out much hope for further movement.

And they could not. With the January changes, the Bush Administration had tried to wash its hands of the travel issue. Even the vanishing prospects for Congressional action and the growing diplomatic disaster were not enough to catalyze further action. A push would have to come from the highest levels of the Administration, and this appeared less likely with each passing day.

The day after our meeting with West and Howard, Ziegler, Volberding, and I remained in Washington to meet with representatives of the 1991 Florence and the 1992 Boston conferences. After describing the organization of our conference, our program plans, and our budget to the organizers of the next two international conferences, we sat down to eat lunch. I was explaining some of the political complexities of organizing the meeting, when, almost on cue, a secretary ran into our conference room saying that I had an "emergency" call from our San Francisco office. I lifted the phone; it was our rather frenetic business manager, whose threshold for the label "emergency" was notoriously low.

"The President's office has been trying to reach you all day!" she panted. "The president of what?" I asked, and was promptly told "of the United States."

9 THE QUICK FIX

Two weeks before our Washington meeting, Dana Van Gorder had spoken by telephone to his friend, *Los Angeles Times* AIDS reporter Victor Zonana. Dana was frankly surprised that in the preparation of dozens of newspaper articles about the boycott, no reporter had asked whether President Bush would speak in San Francisco. After all, we had known that the President was not coming for over three months.

Dana thought the time might be right to break the story. The knowledge that Bush wasn't coming might elevate our political stock in the AIDS community by further distancing us from the U.S. government. Dana didn't hold out much hope that the White House would flinch in response to the heat generated by public knowledge of Bush's decline of our invitation, but it merited a try. The travel issue was stalled. "By the way," he told Zonana, "Bush turned us down."

After Zonana's scoop was published in the *Los Angeles Times*, the White House was asked for comment on the President's decision. Deputy Press Secretary Alixe Glen said, "Each scheduling request is looked at very carefully, and I know that was the case for this one as well. The President, both as a candidate and in his administration, has addressed the AIDS issue and the need for compassion many times." She noted that Bush would be speaking at the National Business Leadership Conference on AIDS in late March, and that Louis Sullivan was considering an invitation to address our conference.

John Ziegler told Zonana, "We're disappointed. We felt this was a real opportunity for the government to make a strong statement." But Ziegler's statement was designed for public consumption. The "Just Say No" committee members were anything but disappointed by Bush's decision. If anything, the security and logistical maelstrom of a Bush visit had only grown in the months since our invitation. When a *San Francisco Examiner* headline described conference organizers as "Miffed by Snub of Critical Annual Conference," our Communications Director Jim Bunn and I went from office to office, looking in vain for the mythic miffed organizer. We found no one.

I had never been called by the Office of the President before, and I found it a rather heady experience. I had messages from two people: Tony Benedi in the Office of Presidential Scheduling, and Alixe Glen, the White House Deputy Press Secretary. I called Benedi first.

"The phones are ringing off the hook," he said. "People are complaining that the President is not speaking at the conference."

"I'm sorry," I said, "but he was invited, and *he* turned *us* down."

"But your letter gave us a reply date of November 30— we can't possibly know that far in advance whether the President can attend an event. You shouldn't have asked us to reply so early. That's why you just got our form letter. If he had been invited later or there was no due date, the answer would have been different."

So we were to be blamed for asking for a prompt response.

I asked Benedi to look over the letter from the White House to see if there was anything that implied that the President might reconsider if asked again later or that encouraged us to extend the response date.

"No," said the White House man, "but most groups will call us back and reissue an invitation if they really want him."

I told him that we obviously had no way of knowing this; the letter appeared to be a fairly unambiguous decline. "We didn't want to be rude. We know how to take no for an answer," I said.

"In any case, the President is very concerned about AIDS and has shown his compassion many times." This was exactly what Glen had told the *Los Angeles Times*—a real, live White House sound bite. So they even talk like this when they're off camera, I thought. "He does not want to be seen as not interested," Benedi continued. "You might consider reissuing the invitation."

My initial shock regarding the caller's locale quickly dissipated. I sensed an opportunity. "To be perfectly honest," I said, summoning forth my innermost chutzpah, "I'm not sure the President would want to have a presence unless the HIV-travel issue is fixed. If he could make a statement of support for a change in the travel policy, then his presence would be most welcome," I continued, hoping that the tremor in my voice was not reverberating through the telephone. "We will consider this and get back to you early next week."

"Fine," he said. "If this travel issue is important, just mention it in the letter of invitation." He concluded by telling me that, if we chose to reissue the invitation, it should be directed to David Demarest, the President's Director of Communications.

My next call was to Alixe Glen, in the White House press office. I knew of Ms. Glen from Rex Wockner, a syndicated reporter whose inquiries had helped fuel this entire episode. Wockner, after learning from Zonana's piece in the *Los Angeles Times* that Bush would neither be speaking at the conference nor sending a videotape, called the White House and asked why. "I spoke to Alixe Glen," Wockner had told me a few days earlier, "and she told me that you hadn't asked Bush for a video." This was simply wrong, I told Wockner, and I read him passages from our invitation letter and the White House's rejection letter. He called me the next day, and told me that the White House had initially misplaced the letters, but now confessed its error.

"Rex Wockner tells me that you and I have been involved in a bit of a misunderstanding," I said to Glen when she reached the phone.

"Yes," she said, "I looked all over the place for your letters and couldn't find them initially. But now I've found them, and there's no question that the President was offered a role and we turned it down. To be perfectly frank, this was a real screwup by his scheduling office. This should have been routed separately, and you should have received a different letter which asked you to hold off on the invitation until closer to the conference. Instead you just got the usual form rejection, which was inappropriate." She went on to tell me the same thing that Benedi had—that the President was very concerned about AIDS and did not want to be seen as indifferent to the issue.

She too encouraged me to resubmit the invitation. I reiterated that it might not be in the President's interest to appear at the conference if the HIV-travel issue wasn't rectified soon.

She rejoined with the party line. "But Congress added that legislation, and they have to be the ones to remove it."

"I've spent the last two days meeting with representatives from the Public Health Service, State, and Justice," I said, "and it's pretty clear to us that a few words from the President would lead to a prompt solution to this problem." Like Benedi, she encouraged me to say this in the reinvitation letter.

As I hung up, I realized that we had been presented with our best opportunity to change the policy and save the conference from turning into a political circus. Lars Kallings had been listening to my end of both phone conversations with the White House. I asked the IAS president what we should do.

"As you remember, I was against having the President at the conference when we discussed it months ago," he said somberly. "But at this point, if the price of fixing the travel issue is his presence at the conference, I believe that's a small price to pay. The boycott has changed the entire equation."

Over tuna sandwiches, Kallings and I drafted our letters to the President and Communications Director Demarest. Kallings encouraged me to insert a note of urgency into the letters, since a decision by IAS to withdraw on March 9, 1990—barely two weeks away—could start the boycott ball rolling at a speed so fast that it would be unstoppable, notwithstanding later actions by the U.S. government.

We decided to send Bush a bland reinvitation that, once again, asked that he "review the policies your Administration will pursue to meet the scientific, social, and political challenges posed by the AIDS epidemic in the coming decade." But in our package for Mr. Demarest, the letter to Bush was buried under one addressed to Demarest himself.

"Since our original invitation," I wrote in the letter to the Communications Director, "certain aspects of U.S. immigration policy toward HIV-infected people have gained worldwide attention and threaten to cause serious damage to the conference and international embarrassment to the U.S. government." I listed many of the groups and individuals, including Luc Montagnier and polio vaccine discoverer Jonas Salk, who had gone on record as opposing the present policy and were considering a boycott. "The President's prompt endorsement of the elimination of travel restrictions would, we believe, end the boycott and prevent this policy from being the major focus of this year's conference among the participants and the media. . . .

"If the HIV-travel issue reaches a satisfactory solution and the international boycott is cancelled, we believe that Mr. Bush will receive a warm welcome from the conference delegates," I wrote, wondering if it was really true. "If, however, such a solution is not achieved, the President's participation may serve only as a focal point for further international criticism on this issue."

We made a conscious decision to initially keep the press unaware of our reinvitation to the White House, sensing that the momentum was beginning to turn our way. Embarrassing the Administration now would do nothing to speed the process and could potentially incite the conservatives, who would resist any further change in the travel policy. Although the right wing had been uncharacteristically silent, we continued to recognize that a Gallup poll asking Americans whether they favored letting more people with AIDS into the country would yield an overwhelmingly negative response. However, if the poll reframed the question to ask whether an HIV-infected researcher should be able to come to San Francisco for a week to attend the International Conference on AIDS, or a four-year-old child with AIDS whose last wish was to go to Disneyland should be allowed the opportunity to do so (one such child had been denied entry a year earlier), the answers would probably be different. Therein lies the fallacy of public opinion polls—what you get back depends on what you ask.

In any case, our goal was to work behind the scenes in Washington, and the best way to do this would be to enlist the help of the White House Communications Office, which is paid to handle damage control for the President. I hoped my letter to Demarest would convince the Communications Director that, unless his boss acted promptly, he'd be spending the spring cleaning up a mess that could have been prevented.

The IAS meeting on March 9 in Frankfurt had the expected outcome. The organization "strongly condemned" the U.S.

policy and, while recognizing "initial progress" on the issue, resolved that "the IAS will only continue to support the Sixth International Conference on AIDS in San Francisco as long as positive changes continue to be made." So we were safe from an IAS boycott, at least for the time being. The position paper continued: "We resolve that further IAS-sponsored conferences will not be held in countries that restrict the entry of HIV-infected travelers. That means that the Eighth International AIDS Conference scheduled to be held in Boston in 1992 cannot be held as planned unless the present travel restrictions are changed."

The IAS statement, when combined with the European diplomatic boycotts and domestic withdrawals by groups like the Names Project (which manages the AIDS Quilt) and the Gay Men's Health Crisis, demonstrated once again to official Washington that further change was required. In early March, all our contacts in the Capitol told us that the Health and Human Services and State Departments were now strongly in favor of solving the problem. Unfortunately, the Justice Department was uncooperative, contending that a solution was impossible without new Congressional action. Reportedly, Attorney General Thornburgh had stopped returning Health Secretary Louis Sullivan's phone calls on the issue.

To try to move things along, we released news of our reinvitation to the President. This generated a small stir, but it was mostly local. On the front page of the *San Francisco Examiner*: "Bush Asked to AIDS Conference—Travel Restrictions on HIV-Infected Still a Major Issue." "The Administration would like to see a remedy," said the omnipresent Alixe Glen. "Is there a way along with the will to make this happen?" We wondered the same thing, and waited for the White House to parry our thrust.

On March 22, David Demarest, the President's Communications Director, called. Sounding like a man juggling a bushel of hot potatoes, he came directly to the point. "We're working on this thing here, but I need to know what the real problems are. Are they problems of perception or are they problems of reality?"

I explained to him some of the tangible problems posed by the travel policy. The policy would result in real discrimination against HIV-infected travelers. The computerized database held the potential for troubling confidentiality breaches. Moreover, many important speakers would not be coming to the conference because of the policy, I exaggerated—possibly including Luc Montagnier.

The implication of Demarest's question was clear and accurate. In the travel wars, perception loomed as large as reality; the Communications Director knew better than most that the two phenomena are often inseparably partnered. "Two thousand members of the international press will come to San Francisco looking for a story," I told the President's spin doctor in my most foreboding tone. "If the travel issue isn't fixed, then this will be the story of the week. No question."

"The Attorney General's office is telling me that they can't fix it within the limits of the law," Demarest went on. "I'm not an expert on law, but I am an expert on communications. And from that standpoint, I agree that we have a problem here. Who do you have working on this in the Congress?"

I ticked off the few members of Congress who had taken up our cause: Ted Kennedy, Henry Waxman, and our Bay Area Representatives Nancy Pelosi and Barbara Boxer. I was pessimistic, however, about Congress's chances of passing legislation in time to save the conference. "The problem is that this will not be a simple fix," I said, "since any bill in Congress will have to confront both immigration and travel. I have four hundred of the top AIDS experts in the world on my Program Committee. Some might disagree about unrestricted immigration for people with AIDS. But not one of them would disagree about the importance of free travel, and this is not a group of ACT UP members. This is a group of responsible scientists and public health experts."

"We're working on coming up with an administrative order

that might later be challenged, but would last through the conference. How long do you think you would need?" he asked me.

It was obvious where he was heading. An administrative fix would likely be challenged legally in the courts or politically by the conservatives. A Jesse Helms spokesman had made it clear earlier that week that the conservative senator would fight any change in the law. Therefore, the trick was to find an administrative solution that could withstand these challenges for just long enough to remain viable through the conference. I told him that an administrative fix invoked six weeks before the conference, if accompanied by some movement in Congress like the introduction of legislation, would be enough to save the conference and the Administration from international humiliation.

I left one last thought with Demarest. In a week, the President would give a speech before the National Leadership Coalition on AIDS, a group of prominent business executives. Some indication that Bush supported a change in the HIV-travel policy would cause many to rethink their boycott of the conference. Demarest promised to do what he could.

President Bush's speech on March 29, 1990, before the National Leadership Coalition was his first address on AIDS since taking office fourteen months earlier. In the speech, Bush appealed for compassion for people infected with HIV and threw his support behind a bill that would outlaw discrimination against people with disabilities, including AIDS. "We don't spurn the accident victim who didn't wear a seatbelt," the President said. "We don't reject the cancer patient who didn't quit smoking cigarettes. We try to love them and care for them and comfort them. We do not fire them. We don't evict them. We don't cancel their insurance."

The President, claiming that the government was "on a wartime footing" in the fight against AIDS, defended the efforts of the NIH and CDC. "We are slashing red tape," he said. "Accelerating schedules. Boosting research." Urvashi

Vaid, Executive Director of the National Gay and Lesbian Task Force, wasn't buying. Carrying a sign that said TALK IS CHEAP, AIDS FUNDING IS NOT, she interrupted Bush repeatedly through his speech. At one point, Bush paused and addressed the heckler and the audience. "I understand the concern that these people feel. If we do nothing else, I hope we can make them understand that not only you care, but we care, too."

Notably absent from the speech was any mention of the travel restrictions. A White House AIDS adviser said the President did not call for removal of the restrictions because "politically, it isn't worthwhile. . . . If the President were to call for the repeal of something that passed ninety-seven to zero in the Senate, his words would fall on worse than deaf ears. He would just be inviting trouble."

But the event gave us some cause for optimism. Before the speech, Bush met with June Osborn and asked her: "Is there anything else I can do?" Never one to mince words, Osborn quickly replied, "Yes, Mr. President, there is." She then described the HIV-travel issue and its consequences for the upcoming San Francisco conference. Bush listened carefully and said, "I thought that was fixed." Osborn enlightened the President and urged him to issue an executive order abolishing the travel restrictions, and support Congressional legislation to change the policy.

It is possible that the President's surprise was genuine. The overwhelming amount of information delivered to the modern President means that virtually everything he receives is predigested and distilled by his staff, who are thus able to promote their own agendas by presenting incomplete or distorted information ("Oh, the HIV-travel thing. We fixed that weeks ago.")

But there is another, more cynical scenario. Sources told us that Bush, in fact, had been briefed on the travel issue before his speech and was well aware that it was not "fixed." By feigning ignorance and trumpeting compassion, he deflected the inevitable criticism from the AIDS lobby. Old

Washington hands suspected the latter, more Machiavellian scenario, and saw in it the handiwork of conservative White House Chief of Staff John Sununu. If so, it would not have been the first time that Bush and Sununu put on their good-cop, bad-cop hats. "The two play off each other like a wrestling tag team on late-night cable: Gentleman George and Snarlin' Sununu; the King of Kind and Gentle and his Dark Prince," wrote *Time* magazine in May 1990.

It was Sununu, in fact, who had persuaded the President to deliver the AIDS address. A few days earlier, reacting to reports that activists would try to interrupt the address, Bush petulantly told his aides: "Well, then I just won't give the speech." Sununu raised his eyebrows and said, "This, from the man who braved the drug lords of Cartagena?"—referring to Bush's macho trip to Colombia. Bush laughed, and agreed to give the AIDS speech.

Bush's failure to address the travel issue in his speech provided the impetus Congress needed to act. "Today was D-day for the Administration to do something and they said no, so the ball is now in Congress," said Steve Morin, Representative Pelosi's staffer and a member of our Community Task Force. One week after Bush's speech, a bill was introduced in Congress to give the Secretary of Health and Human Services the power to review and revise the list of dangerous and contagious diseases. The bill's sponsor was a conservative Democrat from Georgia named J. Roy Rowland, a physician and a member of Osborn's National Commission. "The purpose of our bill is simply to give health professionals the authority to make health decisions," said Rowland. "This is the way it was prior to 1987. And if the U.S. is to continue to be a major participant in worldwide efforts to conquer AIDS and other diseases, we should again put the health decision process in the hands of health professionals."

Morin called us to announce the bill's introduction. The game plan was to move the bill quickly through the House of Representatives, and then debate it in a House-Senate conference committee, thereby avoiding the Senate floor and Helms's porcupine power. The long-awaited introduction of the bill was a cause for celebration in our office.

The celebration lasted for just an hour, when Morin called back. His voice filled with bewilderment, he told us that, though the White House was tacitly encouraging the legislation, Kay James, spokesperson for Health Secretary Louis Sullivan, had blurted to Phil Hilts of the *New York Times* that "we cannot support the bill in any way, shape, or form."

We shared Morin's shock. After working for months to fashion legislation to give the Secretary of Health the power to remove HIV from the list, and being given every indication from Washington that the Secretary and the White House would be supportive, or at worst noncommittal, we were dumbfounded to learn that Sullivan now opposed the bill. I quickly called the White House and spoke with Hans Kuttner, assistant to domestic policy advisor Roger Porter, and the architect of the White House AIDS policy. Kuttner was also surprised. "She [spokesperson James] overstepped her bounds. She will call the *Times* back and change her statement." And that's exactly what she did, although the story in the *Times* the next day highlighted the Administration's disarray. "As White House officials were cautiously backing the bill," wrote Phil Hilts, "officials speaking for Dr. Louis Sullivan . . . said, 'We do not support this legislation.' Later in the day they tried to retract the statement, but finally said they could not decide what statement to make."

Representative Henry Waxman was as astonished as we were. "I don't understand," said the California Democrat who cosponsored the Rowland bill. "Last week, the White House said it didn't have this authority. This week they are saying they don't want it. Either they are in total confusion or they just don't want to decide."

*   *   *

The Administration's Alphonse and Gaston act was a large nail in the Rowland bill's coffin. Congress was not about to give the Health Secretary authority he seemed not to want.

The final nail was driven in when publicity over the gaffe alerted the right wing to the behind-the-scenes activity surrounding the HIV-travel issue. In April 1990, Jesse Helms opened his yawning maw:

"Is it not enough that the public health agenda of America has been torn apart by the AIDS movement," Helms told the full Senate, "and that innocent children—like Ryan White—continue to die because the lobby and its allies promote civil rights rather than public safety? Apparently not, because some in the Administration are bowing to the incessant cries of the homosexual rights movement to throw open the floodgates which our sensible immigration restrictions have previously kept shut."

With Helms aroused, Demarest and his administration cronies found themselves in a political predicament. They needed immediate action to stem the criticism from Europe and the domestic AIDS lobby. Finger-pointing at Capitol Hill would no longer suffice, since the Administration itself had fumbled away any chance for prompt passage of the Rowland bill. Our only hope lay in David Demarest's "administrative fix" to be invoked six weeks before the conference. Christmas—Good Friday, actually—came three weeks early.

When the Justice Department's travel plan was announced on Friday, April 13, details were a bit sketchy. But that was understandable, since the details were yet to be finalized. Earlier in the week, sources told us, the White House Domestic Policy office had called officials at State, Justice, and Health and Human Services and simply said, "Fix it."

According to the new plan, individuals attending a conference preapproved as being "in the public interest" and planning an American stay of ten days or less would not need to answer Question 35 (the "dangerous and contagious diseases" question) on the visa application as it pertained to HIV infection. I guess we should have been flattered, since our conference was the first to be designated by Health Secretary Sullivan as being "in the public interest." In other words, if the applicant was an infected conference-goer, he could answer "no" when asked if he harbored a dangerous contagious disease. The transparency of this legal fiction was lost on no one. The infected individual would still require a ten-day waiver, and those asking for such a waiver were probably infected. But the individual would not be coerced into declaring his HIV infection status; thus the status could not be recorded in official documents or databases.

Although reaction from the AIDS lobby was predictably negative (Merv Silverman called it a "minus two on a scale of one to ten"), most of the weary combatants acknowledged that the long fight had come to an end. The conference was simply too close, and there were too many other issues to tackle. Still the question lingered: Why had the Administration not done more? By making its April 13th change, the Administration had proved false its oft-repeated assertion that it lacked the power to modify the restrictions. That it could authorize special waivers for people attending our conference for ten days meant that it could do the same for *any* conference or *any* length of time.

The timing of the announcement helped answer the question of why Bush had not done more. The announcement came late in the afternoon on Good Friday, timed to reach the generally ignored Saturday newspapers in the midst of a long holiday weekend. Reporters interested in bird-dogging the story found that official Washington had closed up shop. We guessed that the intent of the unusual evasion of publicity was to diminish conservative ire.

Further credence for this thesis came with a Justice Department briefing document entitled "Questions Likely to Arise Regarding the Waiver for HIV-Positive Aliens." Surprisingly, the questions in the booklet represented not gripes anticipated from the AIDS lobby but those anticipated from the conservative flank: "What is the possible legal justification for [the new waiver policy]? Wouldn't a legislative response be more appropriate in light of the questionable legal basis of the administrative action? Why should anyone care whether the [San Francisco] conference takes place?"

The changes had Demarest's imprint. This was the "short-term fix" that he hoped would withstand a conservative challenge until after the conference. Once again, the Administration had readjusted the mix in the policy brew, searching for perfect equilibrium. This time, though, its alchemy worked. The conservatives squawked, but since the Helms Amendment remained the law of the land and would be fully enforced once our conference tent folded, their challenge to the Good Friday fix was perfunctory. And though many community-based and PWA organizations, especially in Europe, denounced the changes, they were sufficient to allow the IAS, WHO, and major AIDS scientists (including Montagnier) to begrudgingly announce their intention to come to San Francisco in June.

I was not surprised when in late April the White House called once again to say that President Bush would not be coming to the conference. As before, we were not disappointed. The White House's request for the reinvitation had provided the opening we needed to move the Administration on the travel issue. Bush's actual presence was no longer necessary.

In the end, the travel issue had given us an opportunity to distance ourselves from Washington and the Bush Administration—a chance to create Jonathan Mann's "international zone" in which the conference program would not be trashed as an Administration mouthpiece. Ironically, the highly politicized travel issue had provided our best hope for depoliticizing the conference.

But politics could not be completely extirpated from the proceedings. Bush would not be in San Francisco, but his stand-in was almost guaranteed to catch hell for the travel issue and other unpopular Administration policies. In early May, we learned that the stand-in would be Dr. Louis Sullivan, who accepted our invitation to speak at the closing ceremony.

"Serious thought was never given to Bush attending the gathering that is expected to attract twelve thousand people," wrote AIDS reporter Laurie Garrett in *Newsday*. "Even a video, said an official who asked to remain unidentified, 'was sure to be booed and jeered, tomatoes thrown, the whole works' by activists angry at federal immigration policies. . . . The highest ranking official at the conference will be Louis Sullivan. 'And that's adequate,' said Alixe Glen."

10 THE AIDS IRGUN

Although I slept better at night knowing that the President would not be coming to the conference, I was not completely reassured. As the winter of 1990 turned into spring and the travel issue played itself out, our attention turned increasingly to the threat of violence.

By spring, Larry Kramer's colleague, film historian Vito Russo, had accepted our invitation to speak in the opening ceremony. Russo's health was failing; we fervently hoped that he would be well enough to come to San Francisco since he was uniquely suited to help the world understand ACT UP's perspective. "Remember that some day the AIDS crisis will be over," Russo once said in a speech. "And when that day has come and gone there will be people alive on this earth—gay people and straight people, black people and white people, men and women—who will hear the story that once there was a terrible disease, and that a brave group of people stood up and fought and in some cases died so that others might live and be free. I'm proud . . . to be part of that fight."

But Larry Kramer remained strangely and uncharacteristically silent. After the "Uncle Tom" letter of December 1989, and a few conversations related to the conference program

(I had invited him to speak in the session on activism and, surprisingly, he accepted), I didn't hear of or from him until March. He was a nonplayer in the travel imbroglio. But like the clock whose ticking is noticed only by its absence, Kramer's silence was conspicuous—and ominous.

My in-laws, liberal New Jerseyites, struck up a conversation with a New York ACT UPer at a party in mid-March. When they told him what their son-in-law did for a living, he asked if I'd seen Kramer's monthly column (aptly entitled "Kramer vs. . . .") in *OutWeek*, a New York gay publication. I hadn't, and so they forwarded a copy to me, with the ACT UPer's handwritten message penned above the article's title, "A Call to Riot." "I hope that when Larry and I say 'riot' or . . . 'burn down the Moscone Center,'" wrote my in-laws' new friend, "[you understand that] we are using hyperbole to emphasize the massive, angry nature of the San Francisco protests. AIDS activists will not depart from our history of nonviolence—we stand for saving lives, not endangering them." His words were inadequate to sweeten the taste of Kramer's bitter medicine.

"Every human being who wants to end the AIDS epidemic must be in San Francisco from June 20–24, at the Sixth International Conference on AIDS, either inside or outside the Moscone Center, or the Marriott Hotel, screaming, yelling, furiously angry, protesting, at this stupid conference," Kramer wrote in *OutWeek*. After venting his spleen against the AIDS Clinical Trials Group (ACTG), the NIH consortium that tests new AIDS drugs, he continued:

> The same Doctor Strangeloves who control the ACTG system are the same Doctor Strangeloves who are controlling the agenda of, and shutting out any dissident voices from, the Sixth International Conference on AIDS. . . .
>
> This conference is going to be about as "Interna-

tional" as the Ku Klux Klan. . . . Any foreigner who
has AIDS or is HIV-positive and wants to come to the
"International" AIDS Conference is forbidden entry
past our Statue of "Liberty" . . .

In other words, THE SIXTH "INTERNATIONAL"
AIDS CONFERENCE WILL BE A SICK JOKE. . . .

THE STRAIGHT WHITE MAN IS THE GAY PER-
SON'S ENEMY! HAVEN'T WE HAD ENOUGH
PROOF? HOW MUCH MORE EVIDENCE DO YOU
NEED? DO YOU HAVE TO BE LINED UP IN
FRONT OF A FIRING SQUAD BEFORE YOU
FIGHT BACK?

*WE HAVE BEEN LINED UP IN FRONT OF A
FIRING SQUAD AND IT IS CALLED AIDS.*

WE MUST RIOT! I AM CALLING FOR A FUCK-
ING RIOT!

What motivated this diatribe? Did Kramer sense an unparalleled media opportunity that might be overlooked by a
gay community complacent after some recent successes? Or
were these words born of a wounded ego, still bitter after
having been passed over for the starring role in our opening
act?

In a 1987 speech at the Waldorf Astoria in New York, at
which Kramer accepted an award from the Human Rights
Campaign Fund, there was disquieting evidence that he meant
his words to be taken literally. "In a desperate struggle to
secure their new homeland, the Jewish people in Palestine
fighting to establish Israel had an organization called the Irgun. It was an underground guerrilla army, and its members
were extremely disciplined and daring. They started fires.
They threw bombs. They kidnapped. They assassinated. They
executed their enemies. They won. . . .

"We are such passive people, we gay people. We take all

the shit they lay on us and then we lie down and take some more."

But in his 1989 book *Reports from the holocaust: the makings of an AIDS activist*, Kramer provided clues that his motive might simply be to stir the cauldron. "It . . . is controversy that helps an issue stay before the public," he wrote, "so that more people join in debate, in the process becoming, one hopes, politicized." Perhaps Kramer's polemic was just hyperbole, a siren beckoning the masses to political action.

Who was the real Larry Kramer—the savvy media manipulator or the budding terrorist?

This question was answered a month later, in Kramer's April 1990 interview with Marilyn Chase of the *Wall Street Journal*. "It hurts me to say I think the time for violence has now arrived," Kramer said. "I don't personally think I'm the guy with the guts to do it, but I'd like to see an AIDS terrorist army, like the Irgun which led to the state of Israel."

Before Chase called Paul Volberding for comment, Paul and I had discussed how to deal with Kramer's threats in the media. "We have to keep emphasizing the importance of the program—that massive disruptions will get in the way of the dissemination of scientific information," I told Paul, reemphasizing our party line. Paul tried this, but found it made for rather disjointed conversation. "It wasn't too smooth," he said of his *Wall Street Journal* interview. "Marilyn Chase said 'Kramer's calling for acts of terrorism at the conference,' and I said, 'That may be, but we sure have a great program!' "

A more realistic hope for us was that the mainstream activist community would repudiate Kramer, and much of it did. Kramer had gone too far for almost everyone. "Our policy is nonviolent, peaceful demonstrations," said ACT UP spokesman Alan Beck. "We may stage sit-ins to stop proceedings, but we'll have nothing to do with [rioting]." "Violence isn't pragmatic," agreed Robert Bray of the National Gay and Lesbian Task Force. "We decry it."

But the media smelled a good story and egged the activist on. In April and May, Kramer popped up everywhere—interviews in straight and gay newspapers, appearances on *Geraldo* and local TV and radio talk shows. He reacted to the backlash from his own community with predictable sarcasm. "I'm sorry my recent call for riots at the Sixth International Conference on AIDS has upset you," he wrote in an "Open Letter to San Francisco" in the *Bay Area Reporter*. "You are free not to riot and you are free to criticize my call to riot, and I am free not to comprehend your criticism.

"And we are all free to die."

Kramer had exposed a deep divide within the activist community. Though many criticized him for going too far, others agreed that the time was right for direct action. We did not know how many might join Kramer's "Irgun," but a single soldier could change the face of AIDS irreparably. I asked Allen White of the *Bay Area Reporter* whether there were others who shared Kramer's sentiments. "There are many people that feel that something needs to be done to get everyone's attention," he said. "I'm sure a lot of people were inconvenienced in Chicago in 1968, but you can make an argument that the protests there led to the end of the Vietnam War."

The analogy gave me a chill. The call for riot was not going to evaporate simply because moderate gays counseled calm. Our focus turned to security, where it remained until the conference.

Jack Ballentine and Al Casciato, two San Francisco policemen with long experience in dealing with the gay community, had guarded the Pope in his high-visibility 1987 San Francisco pilgrimage and helped secure the 1984 Democratic National Convention at the Moscone Center. But so had everyone else we interviewed for the position of conference security consultant. It seemed that if you had had anything to do with security in the 1980s in San Francisco, you'd done the Pope and the Convention. I wondered if we would soon be added to that elite company, so that the security consultants of tomorrow would say they "guarded the Pope, worked the Convention, and survived the Conference."

Ballentine and Casciato's sensitivity, sophistication with the issues, and unfailing senses of humor got them hired in March 1990. Our security men were spin doctors with badges, convinced that security was best assured by avoiding problems through effective public relations. "We have to be seen as the underdogs," was Ballentine's first rule. "Sometimes that's unpleasant, because it means we have to stand there and take abuse, but in the end the crowd and the press must be on our side. Always remember the press's approach to demonstrations: If it bleeds, it leads."

Ballentine and Casciato urged us to place a strong announcement in the Advance Program warning that those disrupting proceedings would be dealt with sternly. Even if we chose not to follow through with our admonitions in the heat of battle, they said, the policy would let the activists know that we planned to be tough—a worthwhile strategy. It was stretching credibility a bit, but we also decided to analogize those disrupting the conference to the government's enforcement of the HIV-travel policy.

"The conference takes seriously its goal of ensuring the exchange of information," we wrote in the program. "Just as the conference has been outraged by the threat to this critical exchange of information posed by travel restrictions on HIV-infected persons, the organizers are committed to preventing any threat to the free exchange of information resulting from disruption of its sessions. . . .

"Conference security will exercise all available remedies to ensure the orderly conduct of the proceedings, including ejection of disruptive delegates. . . . Violation of local laws will subject offenders to arrest and prosecution."

Although Ballentine and Casciato projected a tremendous sense of inner calm, they too worried about violence. They were well aware that AIDS activist groups had no history of violent behavior, but there were other groups that lacked their pacifist history. "This conference is so big that you'll attract a lot of the crazies," they said. "The abortion people, the fetal research people, and the animal rights people will probably all be here. It's the animal rights folks you need to worry about." They asked whether anyone was doing AIDS research using animals. "Of course," I replied. When they commented on the coterie of animal rights extremists centered around the University of California at Davis and its large veterinary school, I felt queasy. One day earlier, our most recent major speaker had accepted—a scientist from the University of California at Davis lecturing about AIDS research in animals.

On the other hand, our consultants were relatively unconcerned about the Gay Freedom Day Parade, with its long history of well-organized and celebratory marches. Nor were they worried about an anarchist convention scheduled during conference week. "I went to their meeting last year," Casciato said. "It was incredibly orderly. My guess is that they hire an organizer for one day and then let him go."

Bomb threats were our biggest concern. At a politically volatile event like ours, experts told us, we could count on a handful of bomb scares. In general, security personnel weigh the severity of the threat and the difficulty of clearing the hall, usually deciding not to evacuate but to search and investigate quietly. This almost always proves to be the right decision, but I would hate to be the one to have to make it at the moment of truth.

Soberly, we realized that even our conference office might be a target prior to the main event. We initiated a security system in which all office visitors would be given a lapel badge to wear, signifying that they had been seen and approved by our French-born receptionist, Yann Verle. Therefore, said Ballentine, if you see someone walking around the office with a lapel button, "either Yann's given them the button or they've captured Yann." If someone called with a bomb threat, they told Yann, try to get as much information as possible while you delay the caller and signal for help. They were so certain that we would get many such threats that they told Yann, only half in jest, to tell callers, "I'm sorry, but we can't accept a threat from you at this time. Please call back again later."

Although on some days it felt like we were planning a war rather than a conference, we continued to develop the scientific program. The "Marathon Meeting," at which all four local program committees convened in our offices to determine the disposition of the 4,870 submitted abstracts, took place during four days in March. The meeting was a smashing success, an organizational *tour de force*. The one hundred committee members shared a sense of tremendous excitement and accomplishment as they pored through the research—experts in adjacent rooms discussing AIDS in Kenyan children, discrimination in Brazil, and molecular genetics of retroviruses.

At about 2:00 P.M. on the second day of the meeting, a flushed Yann sprinted into my office. In his thick French accent, he panted, "It's a bumm." "A what?" we said, in a scene reminiscent of *The Pink Panther*. "A BUMM!!" he repeated. Finally, we understood. "A bomb will go off in the building in fifteen minutes," the caller had told him in a deep voice, followed by a click. Remarkably, everyone remained calm, and the fifteen minutes passed uneventfully.

As if we were not paranoid enough, a few days after the bomb scare came a series of computer crashes, indicating infection by a computer virus. Our office teemed with computer experts, poking and prodding, muttering things like "this is an interesting case," and speculating about sinister disorders that might be lurking beneath the surface. One of their first acts was to purposefully infect a computer, then advance the machine's internal clock through April 1 and Friday, April 13, since some viruses are programmed to reveal their truly destructive colors on Friday the 13th and April Fools' Day. Once they were confident that there was no hidden danger, the Silicon Valley surgeons extracted the viruses from our computers and restored us back to business.

The bomb scares and computer viruses, coupled with Kramer's outbursts, made our office an anxious, fearful place during much of March and April. But it was downright serene compared to the hysteria that reigned three thousand miles away in the Washington office of Health Secretary Louis Sullivan.

Secretary Sullivan's assistants called us a dozen times, inquiring about how we planned to ensure the Secretary's safety. That Sullivan would be taking the stage at almost precisely the moment a few hundred thousand gays would gather for the Lesbian and Gay Freedom Day Parade did not allay their concerns at all. I explained that the parade was a festive party, and detailed some of our security plans, including extensive badge and perimeter security and a stage high enough that only a pole-vaulting activist could mount it. They were only slightly comforted.

Surprisingly, while Sullivan's advance men knew vaguely of disruption threats and specifically of the parade, they had not seen Larry Kramer's writings, a fact of which I was unaware when they asked whether I believed violence to be likely. I'd grown so accustomed to Kramer's rhetoric that I blandly said, "Although Larry Kramer from ACT UP is calling for a riot, we haven't heard about anything else."

"Riot!" Sullivan's assistant Greg Ruth blurted. "You should lock that guy up if he's calling for riots."

The idea of locking Kramer up had never crossed our minds, though it was a viable legal option. I had little doubt that the cure would be worse than the disease—there would be no better way of guaranteeing Kramer a substantial cult following in San Francisco. The idea was dropped without further consideration.

Sullivan's assistants were not the only ones who thought our decision to feature the Secretary on Parade Day irresponsible. When Allen White of the *Bay Area Reporter* saw the closing ceremony roster, with Sullivan among the speakers, he dashed to my office. "How can you people have done this?" he exclaimed. "What exactly were you thinking about? You are inciting a riot!"

White's columns in the *Reporter*, a gay paper, are widely read; his reaction frightened me. "You'll be the one inciting the riot if you take that tone in your article," I told him. "If you stay calm, I think everyone else will too." Thankfully, this seemed to register, and his article, entitled "Conference + Parade: Volatile Mix," was less inflammatory than I feared. Nonetheless, it still was not going to assuage the fears in Washington. "Louis Sullivan ... a leading supporter of the immigration laws that have triggered the boycott of the Sixth International Conference on AIDS, will address that group on Sunday, June 24," wrote White. "The speech will occur just as hundreds of thousands of people line Market Street for the annual Lesbian/Gay Freedom Day Parade." Sure enough, soon after the article's publication, Sullivan's office called again for reassurance.

Even the usually unflappable Dana Van Gorder was swayed by White's comments, recommending that we tell Sullivan to cancel his appearance for security reasons, or move him to the opening ceremony. I counseled calm, steadfast in my belief that our overall strategy remained sound. "Remember the lessons of Montreal," I told Dana. "The opening ceremony will set the tone for the entire conference, perhaps for the entire decade." Our opening was virtually criticism-proof, with a strong PWA and activist presence and no objectionable scientists or politicians. Thus, I reasoned, any disruptions there would be seen for what they were—publicity stunts. Our only hope was to keep the activists calm during the opening, convince them of the importance of respecting the scientific information and the "international zone," provide them with a credible threat that disrupters would be ejected, and save Sullivan for dessert.

Of course, I too was concerned about Sullivan's appearance on Parade Day, but thought the timing might prove a mixed blessing. When I wrote to Sullivan's AIDS deputy, James Allen, to reassure him, I did so with the knowledge that my career could be aborted if I had miscalculated. But I believed that it was in Sullivan's interest to be there (to demonstrate his commitment to AIDS) and in our interest to have him, if only to forestall the activists' outbursts until the last day of the conference.

The parade, I wrote to Allen, "by providing another place to vent, may actually lessen the chances for confrontation at the conference sites. Additionally . . . demonstrators and (as importantly) the press may have tired of demonstrations by [the last day of the conference]."

A few days later, Sullivan's assistant Greg Ruth called again. He was still worried. "We'd really like a letter from the Mayor of San Francisco, welcoming Dr. Sullivan to the city and assuring him that his security needs have been taken care of. Do you think you could get us a letter like that?"

We met with Mayor Art Agnos and Police Chief Frank Jordan twice in the months leading up to the conference. Agnos agreed to send a reassuring letter to Secretary Sullivan, and both he and Jordan assured us that our security needs would be handled efficiently and sensitively by the San Francisco Police Department.

The SFPD's record was not inspiring. On October 6, 1989, soon after the ACT UP demonstration at the opening of the Opera, two hundred demonstrators staged a daytime rally outside the Federal Building in San Francisco to protest U.S. government policies on AIDS research. The police presence outside the building was overwhelming and far greater than what would be expected for such a small rally. Many activists sensed that the police were looking for a confrontation. Later that night they got one. The police swept through Castro Street, the main thoroughfare of the largest gay neighborhood in San Francisco, and arrested sixty demonstrators who had spray-painted their bodies on the street to represent people who had died from AIDS. Police aggressively brandished billy clubs, injuring a number of activists. Many speculated that the police were trying to teach the activists a lesson after the ruckus at the Opera.

The Castro mini-riot had led to a police inquiry, a shake-up in the hierarchy, and a new crowd control manual. In the months before the conference, the police held one press conference after another to demonstrate their kinder and gentler style. Batons would now be held against the chest, not in the more menacing arms-extended position. All 1,750 officers on the force viewed one videotape explaining why protestors were angry with the U.S. Government and another demonstrating how the AIDS virus is transmitted. Lea Militello, a lesbian officer, was appointed as police liaison to the community, and a unit of "gay-sensitive" officers (almost all gay and lesbian themselves) volunteered to work within the conference walls.

Still, distrust within the community ran deep, and many remained skeptical of the police department's commitment to nonaggression. This skepticism turned to outrage after one officer, in a television interview, was asked about unsubstantiated rumors that demonstrators planned to throw infected blood at police. "I'm not going to tell you I'd take a gun out and shoot them, but I'm not going to tell you I wouldn't," said Gary Delagnes. The officer was quickly transferred to desk duty and his remarks repudiated. But the damage was done, the flames stoked anew.

The cornerstone of the police department's strategy was the creation of a demonstration area. Although some cynically suggested Omaha as a suitable venue, the law guaranteed demonstrators the right to be within "sight and sound" of the Moscone Convention Center and Marriott Hotel. The police decided to create the demonstration area by closing

Howard and Third streets, two major arteries, for the week of the conference.

No one was pleased with the choice, but there were few options. During the 1984 Democratic Convention, a parking lot measuring one square block stood across the street from the Moscone Center and became the demonstration area. Those present at the time describe the scene with passion: part political sideshow, part television studio, part circus. Unfortunately, this option was lost to us, since the parking lot was now a 150-foot-deep pit that would eventually produce a huge addition to Moscone's capacity. For now, "The Pit" (as everyone called it) produced only nightmares.

The problem was that any demonstration area of sufficient size to accommodate the demonstrators would abut The Pit. The circumference of The Pit was outlined by a rickety wooden fence, fully capable of collapsing under the pressure of a few dozen demonstrators being shoved in the wrong direction. The fence, we assumed, was also flammable. Thankfully, our concerns were allayed by the Mayor and the Police Chief, who assured us that the fence around The Pit would be reinforced by the time of the conference.

We wondered how we could keep the demonstrators within the designated areas. "The demonstrators are there to get on TV," said Jack Ballentine. He described another event he had worked, in which activists were leaving the designated area in random directions, creating a dangerously disordered situation for the police on hand. "So we wound up the police bomb-sniffing robot, and set him off in the demonstration area. The cameras ran after the robot, and the demonstrators ran after the cameras. Instant order."

By May, rumors abounded that large numbers of protestors would jump the barricades and storm the front doors of the Moscone Center or lie across the sidewalk blocking the walkway between the Moscone Center and the Marriott Hotel, our other conference site. I doubted that the robot trick would work twice. There was an underground passage between our two venues, but it was small and unkempt; we wanted to preserve this route for staff and emergencies. Predictably, the tunnel became news.

"Whenever federal AIDS researcher Dr. Anthony Fauci visits San Francisco," wrote *Examiner* reporter Jayne Garrison, "he stays in a charming and secluded bed-and-breakfast inn, his favorite.

> On June 20, during the Sixth International Conference on AIDS, Fauci will bed in the modern and huge Marriott Hotel. He need never see the sun unless he wants to. He can walk to the Moscone Center by an underground tunnel.
>
> The reason: security.
>
> "I've never heard of this at any other medical meeting," said a slightly worried Fauci. "What *is* expected to happen?"

Even the reporters were getting frantic over security. A few days before running the Fauci story, Garrison had called me, claiming that someone on the conference staff had strongly recommended that Fauci not stay in his charming bed-and-breakfast. Surprised, I checked carefully with my staff and quickly reported back to Garrison that no one had told the AIDS czar that he shouldn't stay at his favorite inn. "Dr. Fauci is a very important person," I said, "and he can stay wherever he wants."

"Are you claiming that Dr. Fauci is *lying*?" she challenged.

Having begun this venture completely naive about the press, I had learned—with some notable exceptions—to control and enjoy my interviews. I found most reporters to be pleasant and interesting, though harried, and was continuously amused by the smoke and mirrors used by the television version of the beast. After seeing one reporter elegantly dressed in formal shirt, tie, and jacket on television, it was entertaining to see that he wore jeans and sneakers to complete the outfit. The camera simply never panned below his waist. Another reporter spent forty-five minutes setting up a VCR player so he could capture five seconds of me watching a replay of a Larry Kramer TV diatribe and "spontaneously" reacting. (I've since forgotten why I agreed to this foolishness.)

But I continuously needed to warn myself that the press was not always my friend. Conversational style is necessarily different with the press than in social interaction. In normal conversation, the listener grants the speaker much leeway to express the sum of his thoughts, allowing for awkwardness while appreciating the richness and power of the overall discourse.

In dealing with the press, however, one lacks this luxury. Each sentence—in fact, each set of two or more words— needs to be autoanalyzed for content and nuance, the assumption being that it may appear in a television interview or newspaper article totally devoid of conversational context. Perforce one's words become blander and more stilted, much of the complexity and vitality expunged.

Still, it was worth cultivating a good relationship with the Fourth Estate. It carried more power to disseminate information from the conference than any other player. In fact, in the month surrounding our conference, some five thousand articles about AIDS, the vast majority about the meeting itself, appeared in the world's print press. Predictably, our attempt to satisfy the journalists became its own press issue. A journalist from San Diego telephoned for our reaction to one researcher's statement that ours was a "conference by journalists for journalists." Other journalists telephoned about statements that ours was a conference "by activists for activists," or one "by scientists for scientists." The impossibility of the conference being all of these things simultaneously demonstrated our fundamental dilemma.

* * *

As hard as we tried to steer the press agenda toward the science of the conference, the rampant rumors of violence reported daily in the media spoke legions about journalistic incentives. Stories about scientific advances and prevention strategies might be consequential, even lifesaving, but stories about riots sold newspapers. The tension between the media's focus on mayhem and our security concerns consumed much of our energy throughout the spring.

Remembering Ballentine's rule (if it bleeds, it leads), we wondered about the wisdom of allowing television cameras to film in conference session rooms. We were providing a "host broadcast"—a television feed to on-site journalists and to a satellite for worldwide distribution—of major sessions. Since the host broadcast signal would be of superb technical quality, I surmised that extra hand-held cameras in the rooms would be there for one reason only—to film (and possibly provoke) disruptions. Our Communications Committee, led by Dr. Connie Wofsy, became the site of lively interchanges between the "scientists" (Ziegler, Volberding, and myself), who generally favored limiting the free rein of cameras in the rooms, and the "journalists" (led by our Communications Director and former television reporter Jim Bunn), who argued that by so doing we would be seen as "managing the news," a major journalistic faux pas.

Communications Committee meetings ranged from the volatile—shouting matches over First Amendment rights and journalistic ethics—to the downright hilarious. During one discussion over the management of the press room, Jim Bunn asked, "How are we going to deal with press queries?" Making the most of this unintended double-entendre, Dana barely cracked a smile and said, "That's my job."

Eventually, Bunn and the First Amendment prevailed (in retrospect, the correct decision), and cameras were allowed in the session rooms. This concession further heightened our concerns about disruptions, and highlighted our need for a "first response team" to negotiate with unruly demonstrators and minimize disruption of scientific sessions. Dana was the logical choice to lead the group—affectionately dubbed the "Karma Team"—of community representatives (including members of the Community Task Force) and "gay-sensitive" police officers.

In Montreal, such a team had not been preconstituted, but formed spontaneously to deal with the disruption during the opening ceremony. Its leader, logically, was the World Health Organization's Jonathan Mann, whose soothing presence prevented a bad situation from degenerating into possible arrests and bloodshed. This, and his handling of the Community Task Force, convinced me that he might again prove to be our ace in the hole, an extraordinary mediator to be called in if the Karma Team reached an impasse.

On March 19, we lost this option.

"I wanted to write you directly to inform you of my resignation," began the fax from Jonathan Mann.

"It has become increasingly evident, during the past two years, that a great variance exists on a series of issues which I consider critical for the . . . Global Programme on AIDS, between my position and that of the [WHO] Director-General. These issues include human rights, the role of women . . . , the role of community-based nongovernmental organizations, and the importance of working to ensure that drugs and an eventual vaccine be available to the entire world's population in need. There is an essential difference between the Director-General and myself on the appropriate level of commitment to the HIV/AIDS problem itself."

Mann's dispute with WHO Director-General Hiroshi Nakajima, who since his appointment in 1988 had taken steps to limit the size and autonomy of Mann's program, was well known in the AIDS world, but many were still shocked by Mann's departure. "His resignation is a world tragedy," said

June Osborn. "They cannot replace him. There is no other Jonathan Mann, and I don't know what will happen to that program."

Although Mann was restrained in his resignation announcement, a week later he lashed out at Nakajima in an interview with the French newspaper *Le Monde*. "The Director-General's lack of commitment to putting the world program against AIDS into action has become a fundamental issue for me," Mann said.

He told the French paper that he was particularly concerned about discrimination against AIDS sufferers and the need to ensure that expensive treatments were available to the needy. "A hundred times I begged the Director-General to act on these issues. There was never, ever, ever, any reaction.

"Coming at a time when AIDS is still spreading, this kind of attitude completely paralyzed our efforts."

Soon after tendering his resignation, Mann wrote me to withdraw from the conference. I asked him to reconsider: Even without his WHO title, we and the world remained indebted to, and respectful of, his accomplishments. We were committed to his presence at the conference, regardless of the flag he flew under. We finally agreed that he would withdraw from his opening ceremony slot, instead giving a plenary talk on the fourth day of the conference. But we felt obliged to do more. "We'd like to present you with an award at the conference's VIP dinner on Saturday night," I said. Clearly touched, he accepted.

The next day, I received a call from a high-ranking WHO official who worked with both Mann and Nakajima. "The Director-General would like to speak in the opening ceremony," he said. I remained adamantly opposed to politicizing the opening. "I'm afraid I have no more slots," I said. It was only partly true. "How about five minutes in the closing ceremony?"

When he accepted, I realized that Sunday's closing ceremony, with Sullivan and Nakajima, was turning into a political quagmire. After emerging triumphantly from his power play with Jonathan Mann, Nakajima's popularity in the AIDS community was nonexistent. But friends at the WHO told me Nakajima was intent on repairing his reputation in the AIDS world, and wanted to make a strong statement on HIV travel. He was not to be dissuaded.

"I understand there is a VIP dinner on Saturday night that Dr. Sullivan is attending," the WHO official continued. "Dr. Nakajima will be there too."

Our elegant VIP dinner, designed to honor AIDS scientists, policymakers, and community leaders from around the world, had become Dinner at Dunkirk. Jonathan Mann and the Director-General would be seated in the same room, probably for the first time since Jonathan's unceremonious departure from the WHO. To make matters worse, we would be giving Mann an award. I was troubled, to say the least.

John Ziegler, with characteristic optimism, saw an opportunity. "Perhaps we can give them both an award and ask them each to make a short speech of reconciliation. This could be a win-win situation."

Thinking that the bad blood probably ran deep, I was skeptical but willing to give it a try. The next day, I spoke again to the WHO official. "I should let you know that Mann will be at the VIP dinner." (I was too cowardly to mention the award.) "Perhaps this could be a time for reconciliation," I chimed optimistically.

"These are two individuals who will almost certainly go to their graves without having reconciled," came the glum voice from Geneva. "I think it would be all right if they were both at the dinner, but I wouldn't seat them next to each other, and I certainly wouldn't give either of them any sharp utensils."

In the end, the dinner was delightful, and Mann accepted his award with grace and dignity. And, as expected, his speech at the San Francisco conference was moving and powerful.

"In the 1980s," Mann told an audience of five thousand,

"in confronting AIDS, no one set out to make a revolution. Rather, people have only tried—as best they could—to do the work of preventing HIV infection, caring for the infected and ill, and linking national and international efforts. Yet, in carrying forward this work, the deficiencies of our health and social systems have been so starkly and painfully revealed that the pre-AIDS era paradigm of health—its philosophy and practices—have been challenged and found to be desperately inadequate—and therefore fatally obsolete. . . .

"Only ten years ago—it seems a century—who could have predicted what we have experienced, who could have imagined the particular forms of courage and creativity we have witnessed, and who would have had the audacity to think that AIDS would not only mirror, but would also help shape, the history of our time? . . .

"Now, in San Francisco, we face the uncertain years to come. Our solidarity must not desert us now. Here, in the city where the United Nations charter was signed—in this city of special honor in the global struggle against AIDS—we recognize and thank those who have taught us, in their lives and in their deaths, about the power of their love; here we honor those who have guided us as we seek to understand and express the kind of love we call solidarity."

Filled with emotion, I rose with the rest of the audience to salute Jonathan Mann with a standing ovation.

As May became June, my pulse quickened with the pace of events. Each day was a kaleidoscope. While putting the finishing touches on the enormous program—more than twenty-five hundred presentations were planned—we fretted by turns about preventing terrorism and maintaining social grace. Thankfully, the travel issue and the boycott remained background issues, largely dormant since the Good Friday changes. I should have guessed that the respite would be temporary.

With all of the debate regarding the Helms amendment,

we had overlooked an even more draconian law. The Immigration and Nationality Act of 1952 barred individuals with "psychopathic personality, sexual deviation, or mental defect" from entering the United States. In 1967, the U.S. Supreme Court ruled that Congress, in writing the law, intended for homosexuals to fall within this category of exclusion.

Until 1979, the Immigration and Naturalization Service (INS) referred incoming aliens thought to be gay to an officer of the Public Health Service (PHS) for medical examination. If as a result of the exam the officer concluded that the alien was homosexual, he provided the INS with a certificate allowing the immigration agency to exclude the foreigner.

In 1979, after the American Psychiatric Association ruled that homosexuality was not a medical disease, the Surgeon General ordered PHS personnel to stop issuing the certificates. A 1983 Ninth Circuit U.S. Court of Appeals ruling held that the INS could not exclude gays unless such a certificate was issued by a PHS officer, effectively precluding the INS from excluding gay aliens from states within that court's jurisdiction: Alaska, Arizona, California, Hawaii, Idaho, Montana, Nevada, Oregon, and Washington. The INS could invoke the law in other states, but had avoided doing so since 1979.

In the 1980s, the Ninth Circuit's ruling had been tested only once, when, in 1985, the U.S. District Court in San Francisco ruled that the INS could not exclude a gay who wanted to attend the Lesbian/Gay Freedom Day Parade. Although the outrageous law remained on the books, gay groups chose not to challenge it as long as it was never enforced.

All was status quo until June 3rd, 1990, when an extraordinary article appeared in the *New York Times*. "As AIDS Talks Near, Agency Will Use Dormant Law to Bar Homosexuals," trumpeted the headline. Philip Hilts of the *Times* had obtained a copy of a May 22 memorandum from Dr. John West, a West Coast regional PHS health administrator, to his boss, Dr. James Allen. "I want to alert you to a potentially sensitive matter which relates to the Sixth International Conference on AIDS in San Francisco and will affect public perceptions of PHS," wrote West. "Today this region was requested by the Centers for Disease Control (CDC) to make available a PHS medical officer to conduct examinations of aliens who enter the U.S. . . . and who self-profess to be homosexuals. . . . Apparently the INS made such a request to CDC in anticipation of the influx of aliens to the AIDS conference in San Francisco. . . .

"Although this request from INS, in and of itself, does not represent an HIV-specific matter, it is impossible to extricate it from HIV issues. . . . I continue to be extremely concerned about . . . PHS participation in the conference . . . and about security relative to the potentially volatile San Francisco environment during the conference."

According to West's staff, his PHS regional office had been contacted by the CDC and told of INS's plan to enforce the law. But why was the INS shaking the dust off this inflammatory law so soon after making concessions on HIV travel? The answer, according to Hilts, was that INS officials claimed to have been told that some gay groups from abroad planned to test the law by declaring themselves homosexuals when they arrived in the U.S. on their way to the conference. Although not in the habit of asking people about their sexual orientation, the INS made it clear that it would respond if challenged. "If the inspectors get a guy who is coming into that conference and he wants to make . . . that kind of proclamation at the border, the inspectors have no choice," said INS spokesman Duke Austin.

Just who were these foreign gay rights groups who planned to challenge the law? No one—not us, not ACT UP, not the CDC and not the INS—seemed to know.

And why had the INS made such a request to the CDC based on such skimpy evidence of an upcoming challenge? Well, they hadn't, according to the INS's Austin. "The INS made no such request to the CDC or anyone else," said Austin. "The INS had no role or motive in making such a request. We've spoken with the CDC and Mr. Hilts, and they don't know how this story originated."

Finally, why had Phil Hilts, by printing such a provocative story in the *New York Times* less than three weeks before the conference, created an issue when, in fact, there was none? Hilts would later say that he had been misled by Austin himself, who had intially confirmed the INS's concerns about a gay challenge before issuing his later denials. The whole episode was a morass, and only one thing was certain: The story stoked the dying embers of passion over travel.

As the eyes of the world turned to San Francisco in early June, so many new problems were thrust at us that ones like these—ones we thought we had laid to rest—were the toughest. Our plates were more than full, and we simply lacked the time to backtrack and fix problems already dealt with. But that is how we spent much of the month. Our next backtrack led us into The Pit—the deep, potentially dangerous excavation across from the Moscone Convention Center.

My daily commute took me past the Center. One day as I waited for the light to change, I absently viewed the flimsy fence separating Third Street—one of the designated demonstration areas—from the 150-foot fall to the concrete floor of the Moscone expansion. I looked at my watch: the date was June 7; the conference was less than two weeks away. Although this "fix" was supposed to have been completed more than a month previous, there was no sign of impending work to shore up the fence. My mind replayed the horror of the riots at the English soccer matches, and fast-forwarded to an image of hundreds of our demonstrators—the ones we were encouraging to protest outside so that the flow of scientific information would not be impeded—being pushed through the fence and falling to certain death in The Pit.

Later that afternoon, we attended a meeting between police and city contractors. The latter, taking their cues from San

Francisco's Chief Administrative Officer Rudy Nothenberg, were panicked that their work on the Moscone expansion would be delayed by police and demonstrators around the conference area, delays that would cost the city tens of thousands of dollars. But there was no discussion of any remedial work on the fence. John Ziegler asked when we could expect reinforcement to begin.

"I'm from the city," said one of the contractors sitting in the front of the room. "There won't be any work. The fence should be no problem."

We were flabbergasted. The fence was a joke, and we had been assured by the city's top brass that it would be fixed. "We think there is a problem," objected Ziegler, but the agenda moved on. We left in stunned silence, knowing that if people were going to be critically injured at our conference, it would likely be by falling through the fence. It was preventable, and absolutely not tolerable.

The problem, we learned, was fiscal and political. The police fully agreed that the fence needed reinforcement, but lacked any budgetary authority to fix it themselves. Such authority resided with Administrative Officer Nothenberg, and he was loath to spend money for this purpose. We had to do something.

Dana called the Mayor's office and let his press secretary know that we would be leaking a story to the media in a few days about the city's decision to endanger lives by not securing The Pit. Simultaneously, we wrote to Nothenberg to show him we meant business:

"The security of delegates to the conference is of paramount concern, and the conference has taken comprehensive measures to assure their safety," we wrote. "The conference, however, cannot protect the public from hazards on city property. . . . [We] join the San Francisco Police Department in strongly urging your office to take immediate steps to assure the safety of the public. . . ."

Our not-so-subtle strongarm tactics worked. A few days

later, a 1,100-foot wire mesh fence went up around The Pit. The city was $18,000 poorer, but the hazard of The Pit had been eliminated.

If felt nice to win one for a change. But our victory with the fence would be pyrrhic if Larry Kramer's army came to town with guns blazing.

By June, however, Kramer had become almost invisible. Rumors abounded that he had decided against coming to San Francisco. One version had Kramer dejected by his peers' rebuff of the terrorism strategy. Another version had Kramer being contacted by the FBI, who told him that he would be held directly responsible for any violence in San Francisco.

From a practical standpoint I needed to know whether Kramer was coming, so that I could replace him in the activism session with another ACT UPer if need be. I asked Dana for Kramer's phone number; he scribbled (212) 477-RIOT on a notepad before handing me the correct number. But the activist wasn't home; his rasping voice came on an answering machine. "What have you done to end the AIDS epidemic today?" it said. "Leave your name and number. I may call you back, and I may not call you back."

He did call, and told me that, in fact, he was not coming to San Francisco. His mood was subdued, almost despondent. He had tried to lead, but his community had not followed. "Why every gay person in San Francisco doesn't march on the Convention Center . . . to say, 'We are angry, you are killing us,' is beyond me," he would later tell an interviewer.

"I have nothing against the conference," he continued. "The conference is a wonderful theater to demonstrate in. I'm not saying 'don't hold the conference.' What I'm saying, though, is that there are going to be a lot of idiots making speeches. They're all second-rate people, and they're controlling our lives. They should hear our anger."

11 SHARED GRIEF

On June 19, Conference Eve, I went to a party thrown by Leon McKusick, the gay HIV-infected psychologist who cochaired the Community Task Force. "Get it out of your system!" urged the invitation. "Rub up against famous plenary speakers! Plot and scheme with activists!" The event was dubbed BYOB: "Brag about your own breakthroughs."

When I pulled up to McKusick's Castro neighborhood home, there were two doors available to enter the gathering. Over one door, a sign read RIOT. And over the other door: SCHMOOZE. Thinking wishfully, I entered door number two to a noisy and expectant crowd. I prayed that the week would be as easy.

Several hours later, returning to my room in the shiny new Marriott Hotel, I learned that this was not to be. The hotel lobby was still buzzing with activity from the week's first major demonstration. In a well-planned event earlier that day, about a thousand people had marched downtown to demonstrate at the local office of the Immigration and Naturalization Service. The march was orderly and creative—one man, dressed as the Statue of Liberty, carried a sign that read, GIVE ME YOUR TIRED, YOUR POOR, YOUR STRAIGHT, YOUR

NON-INFECTED. Eight people were arrested as they climbed over police barricades, but there were no injuries.

At about 5:00 P.M., as the marchers made their way back down Market Street toward the conference site, a few hundred broke into a run and stormed into the Marriott lobby, where they shouted slogans, set off smoke bombs, frolicked in the fountains, and engaged in mock sex acts on the leather sofas. John Ziegler calmly looked on. "This is San Francisco," he told a reporter. "Anything goes."

The demonstrators, led by a young ACT UPer from Denver, demanded more free passes for people with AIDS. One ACT UP member said, "this should be a conference for PWAs, not for the press," noting that we had set aside 2,000 free registration passes for the media and 375 for people with AIDS. At about 7:00 P.M., Paul Volberding, Dana Van Gorder, and conference attorney Steve Hurst began to negotiate with the group's leaders, who pressed their demands for more passes. The negotiations moved slowly.

Meanwhile, the situation outside the Marriott quickly grew tense. Some of the few hundred police officers on duty, weary after their long shift at the INS demonstration, pushed for a crackdown; they were simply too tired to wait for hours while activists commandeered the spanking new lobby. Their commanders, aware that the troops needed a rest to prepare for tomorrow's opening day—a day that promised to make this day seem placid—also pushed for a quick resolution to the standoff. So did the hotel's management.

Volberding, Van Gorder, and Hurst, realizing that trigger fingers were growing itchy, convinced the demonstrators to designate three representatives to join them for further negotiations at a site away from the Marriott lobby. The demonstrators reluctantly agreed to the plan, and the activists filed out of the hotel at about 8:00 P.M.

The negotiations dragged far into the night, finally adjourning around midnight. But at our breakfast meeting at

6:30 on Wednesday, June 20, none of our negotiating team appeared. Volberding called. "We've reconvened over coffee and Danish at a bistro in the Castro district," he told us. Jack Ballentine was with them, to thwart any attempt to kidnap Volberding, something we considered highly unlikely, but not impossible given the atmosphere.

As the opening ceremony drew closer, rumor after rumor billowed and dissipated, constantly replaced by the next outrageous report. After the rumor that infected blood might be thrown at police, we heard one describing a kidnapping attempt on Louis Sullivan and another in which infected needles would be jabbed at representatives of the Hoffman-LaRoche pharmaceutical company and Dr. Margaret Fischl of the University of Miami. Our paranoia was in full flower, but seemed justified.

Bodyguards were dispatched for Fischl, Volberding, Ziegler, and myself. I felt exceedingly self-conscious with a 220-pound shadow, who reassured me that he had been in the business of "executive protection" for many years. "Who have you protected?" I innocently asked. "I could tell you, but then I'd have to kill you," was the poker-faced reply. Somehow, I felt better with him around.

A weary Volberding called again in the late morning to say that the conference had agreed to issue a hundred and fifty more passes to PWAs, to be distributed by the Community Task Force after the opening ceremony. The details confirmed, the negotiating summit broke up a few hours before the ceremony was to begin. Volberding, exhausted, returned to the Marriott for a brief rest.

Meanwhile, Hoffman-LaRoche was holding a small symposium on antiviral therapy in an auditorium atop elegant Nob Hill. As the meeting began, a group from ACT UP New York claimed the stage to decry the lack of access to Hoffman's still-experimental agent, ddC. While a few in the audience yelled, "Let them speak," most shouted, "Get out!"

"They have no right to disrupt a scientific meeting," said one New York physician. "If we're not allowed to hear this, we're not going to be able to make any progress."

While the debate raged among the audience, the panel, led by Dr. Jerome Groopman of Boston, simply walked off the stage. "I think you should give us the courtesy that will help people with AIDS," said Groopman in leaving. Not to be thwarted, the panel of scientists reconvened in an offstage facility and broadcast the originally planned discussion via video monitor to the waiting audience.

All this and the conference has not yet begun, I thought as I left the beautiful summer sunshine to enter the Moscone Convention Center.

Moscone's cavernous main hall is enormous, covering more than three football fields. Standing at the back of the hall, the stage was barely visible, but eight fifteen-by-twenty-foot screens would carry the image of the speaker to everyone in the room, a few thousand people in adjacent overflow rooms, another few thousand watching in their hotel rooms, and millions via satellite television. So large was the room that the sound system in the rear of the hall had a built-in delay to synchronize the speaker's words with his moving lips.

By 3:00 P.M., one hour before the start of the opening ceremony, the ten thousand seats were beginning to fill. Hundreds of smiling volunteers—many HIV-infected—ushered in delegates from Burkina Faso to Bakersfield. Two side stages straddled the main stage. On one stood members of the San Francisco Gay Men's Chorus, listening to the prelude being played by UCSF's orchestra, which occupied the other side stage. A stylized picture of the Golden Gate bridge hung above each musical group—symbolizing the bridge between science and policy and, we hoped, between scientists and activists. The Gay Men's Chorus had asked to hang a few AIDS Quilt panels memorializing their members who had died of AIDS, but the managers of the Quilt, the Names Project, turned them down. The Names Project was boycotting the conference.

I knew that if, as in Montreal, we lost the main stage to the activists during the opening ceremony, we might never gain it back. So the five-foot-high stage was rimmed with potted plants, which were there for decoration—and as one more hazard to an activist trying to vault onto the stage. The floor in front of the stage was bare; a carpet began about ten feet from the rostrum. We called the uncarpeted area "the DMZ." Activists would be allowed up to the edge of the carpet, but no further. Immediately adjacent to the main stage on either side were the press pens, each demarcated by a flimsy rope. Although the press had been told that they needed to stay within their designated area should a demonstration break out in front of the stage, we knew they wouldn't. In fact, we were counting on them to intermingle with the demonstrators to provide yet another obstacle to seizing the stage.

The cameramen and reporters had a look of expectancy as they filed into their designated areas. They had received a letter in their press packs that day from Police Chief Frank Jordan. "When an order to disperse is read during an unlawful assembly, please follow the directions of the press liaison officer," it read. Few remembered attending another scientific meeting where they had been instructed on how to behave during a riot.

The police weren't the only people working the press. A few blocks away, in ACT UP media headquarters at the Best Western Americana Motel, media-savvy activists, armed with the new instruments of war—Macintosh computers, fax machines, and cellular phones—produced one press release after another explaining every act of civil disobedience. Scattered around the rooms were six television sets, each tuned to a different news program, as well as urns of coffee, platters of

Danish, and bottles of Pepto-Bismol. The poster on the wall provided the latest grim statistics: THREE AIDS DEATHS EVERY HALF HOUR.

Outside the Moscone Center, in the designated demonstration area adjacent to The Pit, several hundred activists gathered behind barricades and confronted about eighty police officers. A few demonstrators began to climb over the barricades and were promptly arrested. The first person arrested was blind. The ACT UP media liaison on the scene promptly trumpeted this poignant detail of street theater to the gathered press. I saw one police commander—assigned to maintain order within Moscone—visibly fidget after his walkie-talkie blurted "there are a few thousand people heading toward the barricade!"

Inside the hall, the "gay-sensitive" police were highly visible; many sported earrings and more than a few wore ACT UP buttons—their pink triangles vivid testimony to the precarious role they had volunteered to play. Unseen to the delegates were hundreds more police, in full riot gear, sequestered in the bowels of the Moscone Center. Some sat ready on horseback or on motorcycle, while others lounged around playing cards. A few struck up a spirited game of stickball on Moscone's loading dock.

Tragically, Vito Russo was too ill to make the cross-country trip to San Francisco. I had asked Dana Van Gorder to canvas ACT UP for a suitable replacement, and Dana recommended Peter Staley, the twenty-nine-year-old HIV-infected bond trader-turned-activist. Staley accepted our invitation, and at 3:45 P.M. walked into the DMZ and surveyed the surroundings. The opening ceremony would begin in fifteen minutes. Dana, mingling among the activists, had heard a rumor that Staley would invite his fellow ACT UPers onto the stage during his speech. He and I approached Staley, and told him that we knew of his plan. "Don't test us," Dana said matter-of-factly. "It would be a *very* bad idea."

Staley stood for a moment, thinking. Finally, he motioned

for a tall blonde man standing in the media pen to come closer. The man wore a badge that said JOURNALIST. "Tell the boys that they can come up to the edge of the carpet, but not to try to climb the stage," Staley told the man. "Okay, I've done it," Staley said to us, as he turned and walked off.

At 3:55, an assistant ran up to tell me that, at the last second, Staley had dropped off a single slide to be shown during his speech. I sprinted to see it. We simply could not allow a slide laden with obscenities or calling for violence to be projected to the audience. Out of breath, I arrived at the projector and looked at the slide. On it was a photograph of George Bush.

The opening ceremony began.

The audience applauded as, one by one, the opening ceremony party took the stage. John Ziegler, looking nervous but distinguished, approached the podium. He wore a red armband on his left arm.

"Before we begin the program," he said, "we would like to bring to your attention an announcement of particular importance.

"As you know, the conference this year was boycotted by nearly one hundred groups, states, countries, and AIDS organizations in opposition to the U.S. immigration policies that restrict HIV-infected travelers from crossing our borders.

"The conference organizers also oppose the U.S. immigration policy in the strongest possible terms." Ziegler described the recent policy changes, and continued:

"We view this change as insufficient. The existing policy remains discriminatory and medically unsupportable. . . .

"You will notice many of us wearing a red armband. These are worn in sympathy and acknowledgment of those unable to attend because of U.S. immigration policy." As a gesture of solidarity, Ziegler asked the audience to stand for a moment of silence. Chairs banged for a moment as the audience stood in a hush. Said Ziegler:

"A message to President Bush and to Congress from twelve thousand conference delegates to end AIDS discrimination cannot be ignored."

Ziegler's opening set the tone of the ceremony. Our goal: to channel the activists' anger over immigration and other AIDS policies into the words spoken from the podium. The message: We're all on the same side here. San Francisco Mayor Art Agnos, his voice booming throughout the hall, continued the theme.

"Eight months ago this week, San Francisco and Northern California were shaken by a seven-point-one earthquake," Agnos began. "It was called the most costly natural disaster in American history. In the space of little more than thirty days, the President and Congress set aside four billion dollars and California passed a special tax. Everyone agreed to fix the damage and retrofit our infrastructure for the future.

"But where is our retrofit for AIDS?"

The audience roared its approval, and the Mayor continued.

"If history should record that this is the last International AIDS Conference in the United States, it should be because we have solved the epidemic and not because some people played politics with human life."

Next was June Osborn, the boldly direct Chair of the National Commission on AIDS. Osborn donned her half-glasses and nearly disappeared behind a podium that Agnos had towered over. She began to speak. Her resolve—and her anger—were unmistakable.

"I would like to dedicate my remarks to all those who are *not* here: to those we have lost thus far in this dreadful AIDS pandemic and to those for whom the discriminatory effects of the United States travel policy prohibited participation, whether through conscience or through fear. To the absent participants I would like to say how sorry I am, and how embarrassed as an American, that our country whose tradition serves as a proud beacon for emerging democracies, should persist in such misguided and irrational current policy."

To further emphasize the conference's solidarity, Osborn turned her attention to us.

"Remember that our hosts and hostesses are the very same people who have led the way in many of the scientific and clinical innovations that have taught us all to care better for people with HIV and AIDS; and they have been running the longest in this marathon. I am in awe of their stamina! I strongly suspect that they feel an aching kinship with those who chose to stay away.

"Yet I also believe they are motivated in part, as am I, by an awareness that we are only just finding our stride in the race, and that the traumas of the present must be endured and outlasted; for it is our children, and our children's children, who have the greatest stake of all in what we do and how we manage to work together and to learn from each other. So we cannot allow ourselves to be tangled in enervating quarrels, or to be thwarted in our solidarity and resolve by persons with unholy agendas. I respect deeply the convictions of those who are not here; but I am glad to be here and eager to learn."

The lights in the hall dimmed; the "Personal Perspectives on an Epidemic" segment of the program was about to begin. Looking down from the stage, I saw Dana buzzing around the DMZ, and Jack Ballentine and Al Casciato perched in readiness on either side of the stage. Outside the hall, the standoff at the barricade continued. Eighty more people had been arrested. But there was no violence. Yet.

Through the magic of videotape, Mary Corwin, an HIV-infected woman, appeared on the eight huge video screens. Her pretty red hair blew in the breeze of Golden Gate Park. Lovely flowers made up the backdrop. The scene was soothing, comforting.

"I want to see my daughter date guys on motorcycles that I can't stand," she said. "Kids get stupid around the age of thirteen; I want to go through that with her. But there's a knowledge in me that says there's a good probability I won't." She paused, then went on.

"We don't have massive fights in our house any more. We'll argue and get mad for an hour or so, and then it clicks in our head that it's an hour of time."

A rainbow coalition of HIV-infected people followed— Hispanics, blacks, whites—heterosexuals, gays, hemophiliacs— all sharing their thoughts on having AIDS in 1990. Their dignity and passion were palpable to everyone in the audience, many of whom were surprised as their misconceptions were corrected. An HIV-infected black woman from Brooklyn named Sallie Perryman spoke of her late husband, an intravenous drug user who had died of AIDS. "My husband . . . held a full-time job and was a caring and loving man, who contributed to his society and his family. . . . If you are an intravenous drug user, you are perceived to be inherently evil and parasitical, despite what your values actually are."

What impressed many people in the audience was the wholeness of these people living with HIV infection. They were real people, and they carried the whole range of human emotions. There were tears, but also humor. There was anger, but also joy. There was frustration over the inadequacies of the health care system, but also support for the battle-weary doctors in the audience. "I want to thank all the working scientists and researchers who are trying to find an end to this nightmare," said Pierre Ludington.

"I'm not going to cure AIDS," he said. "*You're* going to cure AIDS."

Next on the videotape was Larry Kramer, filmed as he stood in the sunshine of New York's Central Park. On his T-shirt was a quote—"By Any Means Necessary"—from black radical Malcolm X, whose picture was also on the shirt.

"You know what is going on and what is not going on, and yet you refuse to use your voices," Kramer challenged the audience. "You are coconspirators in this plague, though you think you are heroes."

As I listened to Kramer's harsh words—softened somewhat by the moderating views of the other speakers, my eyes kept returning to the T-shirt. Was it simply the uniform of Kramer's one-man terrorist brigade? Or did it represent a more subtle strategy? After all, some historians partially credit the success of the moderate elements of the civil rights movement —personified by Martin Luther King, Jr.—to the rage of Malcolm X and his followers. Many reluctant whites dealt eagerly with King, the theory goes, because they feared that they might have to confront Malcolm X if they did not. Perhaps this was Larry Kramer's agenda.

Leon McKusick took center stage. He introduced himself as a gay psychologist, a cochair of the conference's Community Task Force, and a person living with AIDS. He praised the work of the Task Force, work that had assured that HIV-infected people were well represented in the program. He also acknowledged the hundreds of free passes for HIV-infected people distributed by the conference. Then he turned philosophical:

"It's time we realized and responded to the ongoing toll that AIDS is taking upon all of us, as health professionals, as health care workers, and as scientists. At issue here is grief. . . .

"I contend that a large part of the anger of AIDS activism, that loud screaming and yelling you hear outside, is grief. In this phase of our bereavement, we express our anger. But I further suggest that the cold resentment felt by many scientists and doctors against the activists is repressed grief, unexpressed grief, withheld grief. No matter how rational you are, these are extraordinary circumstances, calling up extraordinary emotions, which may cloud our reason. . . . We all want this thing to end. We all need avenues to express our grief as we do."

And with that, he introduced Peter Staley.

The prepared text of Staley's speech, which was available in the press room prior to his presentation, had a large gap where the first few paragraphs would normally go. After our discussion in the DMZ, I guessed what was to come. Staley began.

"In an effort to bridge the gap that now seems to exist between AIDS activists and you, members of the medical and scientific communities, I would like you to join us in an act of activism," Staley exhorted. "Trust me, you'll enjoy this.

"But first, I would like to be joined in front of this stage by my fellow AIDS activists." Perhaps one hundred ACT UPers ran to the front of the hall, hooting and yelling. As expected, dozens of cameramen fled the press pen to join them. I began to perspire, and noticed Ziegler and Volberding doing the same. The activists stopped at the edge of the carpet, and Staley continued.

"At this moment, there are others, just like us, who are trying to get into this conference, but are being barred by the billy clubs of the San Francisco police. And there are still others like us who are trying to get through customs at the San Francisco airport, but are being detained instead because they are gay. And these same customs agents are under orders to keep a lookout for AZT in people's luggage. If you're found with any, you're put on the next plane out of the country. . . .

"There is a man that could end this insanity with the stroke of a pen." The slide of President Bush projected on the large screens, greeted by more yelling from the activists.

"I ask all of you now—you were asked earlier to stand in silence—we're going to do something different. We're going to stand ACT UP-style. If you believe that the present INS policy barring people living with HIV disease from entering this country is useless as a health policy and discriminatory as well, please stand now!"

The entire audience stood, once again, to loud applause. The ACT UPers in front began to chant. "Change the law! Change the law!" Staley appeared to be losing control, as the chanting continued for a few minutes. "All right," he said. "Okay." He made a Hollywood cut signal across his neck. Finally, the chanting receded.

"I ask you to join us in vocalizing our collective anger. . . . Join us in a chant against the man who has decided to show his commitment to fighting AIDS by refusing to be here today. Instead, he is at this very moment in North Carolina attending a fundraiser for the homophobic author of the INS barriers, that pig of the Senate known as Jesse Helms." (It was true.) "Join us in this chant: "Three hundred thousand dead from AIDS! Where is George?"

Many in our audience, including more than a few of the scientists, complied. I noticed a few federal researchers chanting a line or two, then sheepishly looking around to see if anyone was watching. The chanting went on.

"Thank you," said Staley with a disarming smile. "You can all now consider yourselves members of ACT UP."

The activist cited a litany of problems with the federal response to AIDS, including bureaucratic inefficiency within the AIDS Clinical Trials Group, and the failure of federal drug trials to test drugs other than AZT or to include more than token numbers of women and minorities. The blame, said Staley, lay with George Bush. "President Bush," he said, "we're watching your actions, not your words. Your actions are killing us. Your words are lies."

Then Staley's features softened, his face assuming the contours of a frightened youth. With all the bravado, it was easy to forget that here was a man just entering the prime of his life and confronting his own mortality, forty years prematurely. "I understand that I'm supposed to give a personal perspective on living with HIV," he said quietly. "As you can tell from this speech thus far, I have never been able to view my situation as just a battle between me and HIV. I have always been painfully aware that in order for me to beat this virus and live, I will need a great deal of help from all of you, as well as from my government. Cooperation between all of us is the fastest way to a cure.

"However, recently I've begun to lose hope in our ability to work together to end this crisis. If anything, the gap that exists between all of you and AIDS activists seems to be widening. . . .

"On my side, the level of anger and frustration is reaching such a point that attitudes claiming that all of you are un-caring and in it for greed are now widespread. I'm being taught to hate the 'gang of five' "—five prominent AIDS Clin-ical Trials Group researchers—"without ever having met any of them. My good friend Larry Kramer has been trying to talk me into being an AIDS terrorist!

"Is there any way we can avoid all of this? I'm not sure anymore. I do know that we have judged you at times un-fairly. I believe that many of you care deeply about ending this crisis and that greed is not your motivation for fighting this disease.

"I also know that you have frequently judged us unfairly too. Yes, ACT UP has made mistakes, such as choosing an inappropriate target for a demonstration, or using an offen-sive tactic. Communion wafers come to mind. But let's be fair here. When we make mistakes, what's the fallout? Some people become offended and begin to hate ACT UP. Whereas when the government or scientific community makes a mis-take . . . thousands of people can die. While at times we may offend you, remember as well that, like you, ACT UP has succeeded in prolonging the lives of thousands of people with HIV disease.

"Can we all, before it's too late, begin to understand each other? Will we realize that we share similar motivations? Can we try, at least this week, to bridge the widening gap between us?"

Staley closed by quoting Vito Russo, the man he replaced in the opening ceremony. "Like the unsung anonymous doctors who are fighting this disease and are so busy putting out fires that they don't have time to strategize, AIDS activists are stretched to the limit of their time and energy, putting out fires of bigotry and hatred and misinformation when they need to be fighting for drugs and research money. We need luxury time to strategize the next year of this battle, and we need our friends to join us so we can buy that time. And after we kick the shit out of this disease, I intend to be alive to kick the shit out of this system so that this will never happen again!"

Staley marched back to his seat, clenched fist raised above his head, to a standing ovation from the audience. The ACT UPers in front were whipped into a frenzy, each chant getting louder and louder. This was the moment of truth. Would they make a rush for the stage? Would they continue shouting through the rest of the conference?

About a minute went by—it seemed like an hour—and the eight video screens lit up with the final segment of "Personal Perspectives"—a gay black man named Michael Slocum. "I live in fear of the death of virtually everyone I know now," he said, choking with emotion, "because I've built a world filled with positive people, and its a real tentative kind of world." The activists in the front at first continued their chanting, but quickly recognized that they were drowning out the poignant words of another PWA. One by one, the shouting stopped and the activists returned to their seats. Soon, the area in front of the stage was empty. I heaved a huge sigh of relief and settled back to watch the last speaker on the videotape—a young HIV-infected woman named Carla Abbotts.

"I really would like you to put yourself in our shoes for one moment, and try to imagine the impact on your life if your friends around you—your peers—were dying, or your lovers were dead. I know people who have had seventy people in their lives die. If you can imagine what that would be like—each one of you . . . maybe you could come up with some sort of answer."

But it was not yet over. In the keynote address, the pain and seemingly insurmountable logistics of getting our arms around AIDS in Africa, particularly the problems of mothers and children, were eloquently portrayed by Eunice Kiereini, the stately nurse-midwife and Chair of Family Health for the Foundation of Kenya.

Moved to tears, the tentative, newborn coalition of scientists, physicians, PWAs, and activists slowly exited as the opening ceremony ended.

12 THE FRAGILE COALITION

T he reviews of the opening ceremony were gratifying. "What was billed as a possible riot became something of a lovefest," wrote *Newsweek*, "a ritual of solidarity between those afflicted by the virus and those working to stop it. . . . The activists and the scientists found common cause in the battle against fear and ignorance, as manifest in a U.S. law barring infected people from entering the country. While demonstrators stood outside the Moscone Convention Center chanting their contempt for the law, some of the world's leading AIDS researchers donned red armbands and signed petitions to express the same sentiment."

The next three days of the conference went so smoothly that we could scarcely believe it. It was impressive—extraordinary, really—to see an immunologist from Paris mingle with an epidemiologist from Brazil, an activist from New York with a prevention worker from Uganda. Once the seeds of the coalition were planted in the opening ceremony, they simply grew and flourished.

So smooth were these middle days of the conference that my anxieties over the closing ceremony receded (albeit briefly) from immediate concern. I found myself enthusiastically moving from session to session, allowing myself the mindset of a conference delegate rather than a field marshal.

The activists made their presence known, of course, but did so without impeding the flow of information. When Dan Hoth took the podium, his lips quivered with fear. As Director of the Division of AIDS at the National Institute of Allergy and Infectious Diseases, he was the point man for one of the activists' favorite targets: the AIDS Clinical Trials Group. Although not one of the ACTG's "Gang of Five," he was the gang's leader. His bodyguard stood expectantly just offstage.

About fifty demonstrators—most holding banners decrying the low percentage of women in ACTG trials—walked to the area in front of the stage as Hoth began to speak. Hoth summarized the successes and challenges of the ACTG program, then eyed the silent activists a scant twenty feet away. "The involvement of PWAs and their advocates—when constructively applied," he said, "has already and will continue to make a difference." Hoth finished his brief lecture and left the podium. "Women with AIDS can't wait till later. We are not your incubator!" chanted the crowd fronting the stage—exactly twice. Then they stopped, applauded, and quietly took their seats.

Even Ellen Cooper, the official of the Food and Drug Administration who was called "murderer" in Montreal, felt the new spirit of cooperation. Speaking in a session on the Parallel Track—the recently approved system in which AIDS patients are allowed access to experimental medications before clinical trials and FDA testing are completed—Cooper received warm applause from the activists in the audience. "I knew then that hell had frozen over," said one astonished federal scientist.

Of course, there were issues that continued to generate contention between scientists and activists. By design, we confronted these issues head-on—hoping that all the diverse views in the audience would be articulated on stage, thus eliminating one more motive for disruptions. These controversial sessions were scheduled at the same time as more traditional scientific sessions, on subjects like animal research and basic pathogenesis. The issue-oriented sessions would, I hoped, draw all those with political leanings, allowing the scientific sessions to proceed in an atmosphere of relative serenity.

Friday morning, June 22, was typical. In a scientific plenary session, lecture topics included "Prevention of HIV Infection in Drug Users," "Immune Response to HIV," and "Vaccine Approaches." The latter talk, by Jay Berzofsky of the National Cancer Institute, highlighted the major scientific news of the conference: the increasing optimism among researchers that an effective AIDS vaccine would be available before the turn of the century.

Meanwhile, the issue session was devoted to an examination of clinical trials and drug development. The session was a microcosm of the clash of forces over the most volatile issue in the epidemic. The speakers included a pharmaceutical industry representative, an Oxford biostatistician, a Ugandan physician, the director of AIDS Research at the NIH, the activist leader of San Francisco's Project Inform, the director of New York's Black Leadership Commission on AIDS, and the crusty but venerable editor of the world's leading medical journal, the *New England Journal of Medicine*.

The most telling exchanges took place between Martin Delaney, the charismatic director of Project Inform, and *New England Journal* editor Arnold Relman. Delaney had spent the past year embroiled in controversy over his underground tests of the drug GLQ-223, known far and wide as Compound Q. Early test tube studies of the exotic compound—derived from the Chinese cucumber root and used for hundreds of years in the Far East to induce abortion—revealed striking activity against HIV-infected cells. But it was estimated that standard university-based trials of the drug would take years to complete, and FDA approval years more. The community had grown impatient.

In April 1989, the forty-three-year-old Delaney, working

with community physicians, statisticians, and lawyers, went forward with a plan for "renegade research"—an underground trial of Compound Q. "Already, we were hearing that thousands of doses of Q were being imported," said Larry Waites, one of the physicians involved in the trial. "We looked ahead to hundreds of people taking this very strong drug and dying. We wanted to find out fast whether it worked."

The underground trial was carefully constructed to fall within the letter, if not the spirit, of the law. Patients answered a thirteen-page questionnaire, administered orally in a videotaped session, before being allowed to provide informed consent. The patients themselves brought the drug to the clinic, asking their physicians only to supervise and monitor their treatment. The artifice, it was hoped, would protect doctors from liability lawsuits for administering experimental drugs without FDA approval.

The FDA, upon learning of the trials in June 1989, opened an inquiry to decide whether to pursue criminal prosecution. "We expected an investigation, and we welcome it," Delaney said boldly. "This is the story of how we'll alter the way drug trials are conducted in this country—not only for AIDS, but for all diseases."

Eight months later, the FDA handed down its verdict. The agency's decision to allow Delaney's trial to go forward was hailed as a victory by activists. The standard system for evaluating drugs "is just too bureaucratic and inefficient to address the disaster that this epidemic represents," said Jesse Dobson, who works on clinical trials as a member of ACT UP San Francisco. "We've got to try something new."

But many scientists attacked the ruling as an FDA capitulation to activist pressure. The decision "grants carte blanche for people to do whatever they want to do," said Donald Abrams, Chair of our Social Science and Policy Committee and an AIDS physician at San Francisco General Hospital. "It opens a Pandora's box. And the only people who are ultimately going to be hurt are those we are trying to find an answer for."

As Delaney strode to the podium, he was under immense pressure to report results on Compound Q. He had promised the community quick answers, and had succeeded in co-opting the FDA in his efforts. But, like the university-based trial of Compound Q he criticized as lethargic, he had not released any results since beginning his trial a year earlier. After recounting the promise of community-based research, he showed a slide entitled "Reality, 1990."

"With few exceptions, the community-based research groups are moving slowly," he conceded. "They too have learned the problems that the academic centers face." He described a chaotic arena, with dozens of community groups, each with increasingly bloated bureaucracies, competing for scarce funding. "If all we do with community research is duplicate the ACTG, we will have accomplished nothing except our own self-empowerment."

He turned to Compound Q, noting that the drug was in widespread community use before formal studies had even begun. "The academician says, 'Look the other way. Don't do that. We told you not to fool around with that stuff.' But that's nonsense. We have to address the problem. . . ."

Delaney described his observational study of Compound Q, in which patients' CD4 counts (the most widely accepted marker for HIV disease progression), declining steadily before they began to take Q, showed a small rise after taking the drug. The study violated some tenets of clinical research: Many epidemiologists were quick to observe that the increase in CD4 counts could be owing to other drugs taken by the patients, the psychological effects of taking a compound one thinks might help, or chance variations in the test results. But Delaney proceeded without caveat. "This is the real world laboratory," he said.

"I'm frustrated by being caught between a rock and a hard

place. . . . Many in our community say, you still aren't moving fast enough—we're still dying faster than you're studying." On the other hand, "I know I'm going to be taken to the woodshed by the academicians for having the nerve to break out of the conventions of research. For having acknowledged the fact that patients and clinicians are using unlicensed and unapproved drugs. . . . Those shrill attacks are going to continue—we'll probably hear them here this morning. I don't find our program unethical; I find it extremely compassionate. . . . This is the price for sticking our necks out, for not settling for business as usual. I make no apologies."

"I respectfully suggest that Mr. Delaney read more about the history of medicine," *New England Journal* editor Relman replied haughtily. The activists in the audience jeered. "If he does, he will see that the history of medicine through the ages is replete with examples of all sorts of remedies that were tried by individual practitioners—who believed devoutly in the value of what they were doing based on their own experience. . . . I think that we'll get much more rapidly to where we want to be if we follow the proven methods of science. Ask critical questions, design critical experiments, carry them out quickly and properly, and be rigorous and objective in your analysis. That's the way you get the truth. Let's not go back to black magic at this point." Others in the audience of four thousand cheered.

"Mr. Delaney, you really are irresponsible making such claims without publishing your data," continued Relman. "There's no information about who these people were, how sick they were, how long they were on the drug. Frankly, we can't tell if this is a flash in the pan or something great. And that's not useful to patients at all."

"I'd be pleased to give Dr. Relman our data and invite his review if he in turn promised to publish it," replied Delaney coyly.

"We'd be happy to review any data. . . . But we promise

to publish only those reports that our experts feel are worth publishing. We would apply the same criteria to your studies as we would apply to the studies sent to us from any other source. We play no favorites."

Mark Harrington of ACT UP commented on the new dialogue between scientists and activists evidenced at the meeting. Like Relman and Delaney, they were not always seeing eye to eye, but at least they were talking. Unlike other classes of people, said Harrington, "scientists actually are capable of rational dialogue, and sometimes even change their minds."

The coalition between scientists and activists was not the only one that bore watching. The traditionally gay AIDS lobby was showing some cracks under the pressure of the diverse groups demanding their slice of the AIDS resource pie. Although, as before, a number of gay activists spoke of the urgent need to include women, minorities, and drug users under their umbrella, nongay groups were increasingly finding these protestations unconvincing—window-dressing designed for public consumption.

In the session on clinical trials, Debra Fraser-Howze, the forceful and articulate Director of New York's Black Leadership Commission on AIDS, described the absence of blacks in many trials of AIDS drugs. "It is not out of ignorance that some in our community have not responded to clinical trials—but out of knowledge. The knowledge that some trials are utilizing placebos"—inactive pills whose usefulness is compared to that of active drugs—"and the knowledge that if you are already on the low end of the totem pole, chances are greater that you will wind up on the sugar pill end of this epidemic.

"We cannot afford to set up barriers or wars with one another," she continued. "Everybody is somebody's child. When we speak for our communities, we must speak against no other community. . . . When we start making choices about which of our children is more dispensable in their life cycle than another, then America and the world have failed."

Ironically, as Fraser-Howze spoke, dozens of ACT UPers —virtually all white—filtered through the audience distributing leaflets decrying her commission and its policies. "The Black Leadership Commission on AIDS," said the leaflet, "offers no leadership to African Americans affected by AIDS/ HIV in New York City."

Another session—on community organization and activism—demonstrated the widening rift between white heterosexuals and other groups at risk for AIDS. Jeff Montforti of Atlanta came to speak about organizing parents of children with HIV. "I'm not a Ph.D. or an M.D.," he said. "I'm a D-A-D."

Montforti was a dad infected with HIV himself. His wife was also infected, and he had already lost two children to AIDS. "Dealing with children who are ill is really complicated," he told the large audience. "You don't have the time to rest, because you're always sleeping with one ear open."

"There needs to be a network for parents in each community—as there is in the gay community. I think it's absurd that we can be very interested in one population and just forget about other kinds of populations. Families need the same thing that gay men and women need—they need support." As I listened to Montforti's plea, I was again struck by the political changes wrought by AIDS—a heterosexual parent was asking to be treated more like a gay man.

He recalled the story of Baby Jessica, the little girl who became trapped in a deep well in Texas. A mother he knew wrote to President Bush after Baby Jessica was rescued. The mother was touched by the nation's response to the little girl's plight. "I'm in the same position," continued the letter. "My daughter is in a well, and the well is called AIDS. What scares me is that George Bush is not going to call me, and she's not going to get a whole lot of gifts, and she's not going to get all those cards, and there's not going to be a whole mess of people standing around wishing this child well." Montforti, crying as he finished the story, received a standing ovation from the sympathetic crowd.

But a man from New York City rose to speak. "I have a great deal of empathy for you," he said. "When you decide with others to organize yourselves as a part of the AIDS community, I trust that you will not do so on the basis of a uniqueness of a heterosexual experience of HIV, which would jeopardize much-needed money to the several unique communities of color and the unique lesbian and gay community, both of which have been besieged and ravaged not only by this disease but by tremendous forces of oppression and hatred and bigotry. Welcome to the club.

"I would like you to know that there are hundreds of thousands of young, gay, black, Hispanic, brown, red people who have been in wells, and there's been nobody from the federal government to come and say hello."

Unity was a tricky business, made all the more so by the pervasive sense at the conference that the AIDS backlash was no longer merely a theoretical possibility. The resource pie, it was now clear, could no longer be counted on to expand with every year. The advocates for people with other diseases had begun to learn the game and were competing more successfully for a static health care budget.

One morning during the conference (the ungodly hour was 4:00 A.M.), I appeared on the CBS Morning News, and was asked by reporter Paula Zahn about the equity of resource allocation for AIDS. The real answer—involving the political complexity of the allocation process, the potential spin-offs of AIDS research, the difference between epidemic and non-epidemic diseases—would take far longer than the thirty seconds I had been allocated. So I wimped out with what is commonly called the "B-1 bomber" argument. "We shouldn't be pitting AIDS against cancer and heart disease," I told Zahn. "We should be looking at the whole pie, and decide whether we're spending too much money on the military and not enough on more human needs." Too facile by half, I thought, but short enough to fit in the space. At least it won't offend anyone.

A few days later, I received a tongue-in-cheek letter from an old college friend with eight years of Pentagon service under his belt. "Secretary Cheney asked me to pass along the enclosed note. Don't take it personally. I for one was gratified to hear that the fruits of my success in the international security arena could be used to finance current shortcomings in your profession. Indeed, the entire nation should be especially pleased to know that, in your opinion, the nation's defense, health services, education system, and environment (not to mention the budget deficit) are all in sufficiently good shape that currently budgeted resources could and should be diverted toward AIDS research without any adverse effect on other sectors of society. Good job."

Attached was a bogus note from the Office of the Secretary of Defense. "I'll make you a deal," it said. "I won't treat patients if you don't try to manage the nation's defense." It was signed simply: "Dick."

In ACT UP media headquarters six blocks from the conference, Josh Gamson was pleased. "I'd say things have gone very well this week," said the twenty-seven-year-old graduate student and ACT UP media liaison. "We've been on all the national networks, we're the lead story on local news shows, and Peter Jennings is doing his nightly news anchor from here. I don't think you'd see that kind of interest in a conference that was just science."

Every day saw a new cause and a new tactic. Day Two's protest dealt with the San Francisco model of care, which speakers criticized as crumbling. Demonstrators carried signs reading SAN FRANCISCO AIDS MODEL BUILT ON A FAULT, and showing replicas of dollar bills with bloody handprints. Fifty activists were arrested.

On Day Three, about a hundred and fifty members of ACT UP's women's contingent were arrested after staging a "die-in" that blocked traffic on Market Street for two hours. Their demand: that the government investigate more thoroughly transmission of HIV among women and make new AIDS treatments available to women.

On Day Four, about a thousand protestors took over the downtown branch of Nordstrom department store, claiming the chain discriminates against people with AIDS. The activists stormed through the store's brass-handled doors, scores of photographers in tow, and streamed through the multilevel atrium. Lavender fliers swirled through the air like ticker tape, while the demonstrators beat drums, blew whistles, and chanted: "We're here! We're queer! And we're not going shopping!"

"Sure, they have a right to demonstrate," said one exasperated Nordstrom patron. "But I have a right to shop."

All told, nearly four hundred people were arrested during the week of protests. But the surreal quality of the staged efforts belied the seriousness of the cause. Some activists were arrested three or four separate times. With every arrest, ACT UP media representatives circulated among reporters like guests at a cocktail party. "Does anybody need any facts about the people arrested?" shouted the handlers. "Does everyone have the spellings straight?"

The odd quality was evident from the first march of the week, wrote Michael Specter in the *Washington Post*. "ACT UP's march began at the headquarters of the Sharper Image, the ultra-yuppie gadget house on Market Street," wrote Specter. "Activists with green hair and banners seeking 'Facts on Fluids' and proclaiming 'Queers Have No Fears' lined up politely at the brazed copper counter of the outdoor espresso stand. Coffee blended from 'beans of six countries' sold out first."

* * *

Months earlier, Dana and Paul Boneberg had conceived the idea of a unity march—one in which scientists and activists would march side-by-side—for the second-to-last day of the conference. We were highly skeptical of the concept at the time; after all, the idea was hatched as we were making provisions to deal with threats of AIDS terrorism. But now, on Saturday, June 23, the idea seemed brilliant, an unparalleled opportunity to cement and celebrate the fragile coalition between scientists and activists.

Boneberg and a number of local groups arranged for the community half of the march. For our part, we pledged to deliver the conference leadership and to advertise the event in our daily newspaper and at our morning plenary sessions. But, we told Boneberg before the conference began, if by Saturday the scientists had tired of being jeered at by activists, we couldn't guarantee that any would want to march in unity.

As we lined up outside the Moscone Center at 11:00 A.M., it was obvious from the throng that many did want to march. Dana led Volberding, Jonathan Mann, June Osborn, Merv Silverman, and me as we lined up behind a banner reading DELEGATES—SIXTH INTERNATIONAL CONFERENCE ON AIDS. The picture appeared the next day in newspapers around the world.

Timing was critical. The community group had begun their march at 10:40 A.M. near City Hall. They would arrive at the corner of Third and Market streets at 11:30, where, in a symbolic act of partnership, our group of conference delegates would merge with them into one. "Let's go!" shouted Dana, but John Ziegler had not yet arrived. We waited, as the crowd of about a thousand conference delegates impatiently began to chant. "Three hundred thousand dead from AIDS. Where is George?"

Volberding and I joined the chant. "Three hundred thousand dead from AIDS. Where is John?" Finally, Ziegler arrived, and we were off.

When the two groups met at Third and Market, the heart-felt cheer could be felt through downtown San Francisco and, via the enthralled media, around the globe. "In a scene that seemed to symbolize the convergence of science and politics, the delegates merged . . . with the noisier, more colorful, whistle-blowing demonstrators," gushed the *San Francisco Chronicle*. "The staid-looking leaders of the delegate group began chanting with the other marchers. Ziegler and colleagues intoned, 'We're all in this together. Action equals life.' "

The parade grew as it snaked up Market Street, chanting all the while. Everything was perfect, except June Osborn's ladylike high-heeled shoes, which kept slipping through the subway grates. Jonathan Mann and I each took an elbow, and virtually carried Osborn the quarter-mile to Justin Herman Plaza, site of the parade's rally.

"The apparent divisions between us are not real," Volberding told the crowd of twenty thousand in the plaza. "We hope this unity march is an example of a new era in our fight against AIDS."

"People ask me if there are any breakthroughs," Ziegler said. "This is the breakthrough. The breakthrough is that we're all in this together. Action equals life."

But even in that heady moment, having accomplished something that most had thought impossible, we could see signs of the gathering storm. Tomorrow, Louis Sullivan was coming to town. And some activists were already fretting about the implications of the unity march, of being "absorbed in the AIDS establishment."

"We're losing our hard edge of criticism," said one New York ACT UPer. "AIDS is still killing us. I came here to agitate, not to collaborate. We should have rioted a long time ago."

13 "YOU WILL NOT HEAR LOUIS SULLIVAN TODAY"

Our strategy of saving the major representative of the Bush Administration until the final day of the conference had paid off in droves. Not only did the activists lack targets during the first four days of the conference, but many remained on good behavior to protect their badges from confiscation before the closing ceremony. They were simply too eager to let U.S. Secretary of Health and Human Services Dr. Louis Sullivan know how they felt about the government's handling of the epidemic to miss the grand finale.

Sullivan's advance team streamed into town on Saturday, June 23, to lay the groundwork for their boss's arrival. We and the leadership of the San Francisco Police Department met them in a Moscone back office.

The flow of information was decidedly unidirectional. The Washingtonians wanted to know everything about our plans for the closing ceremony, but told us little of theirs. Sullivan will be here, they said, but we can't say when he'll arrive or where he'll be staying. They also wouldn't tell us whether he'd attend the entire ninety-minute closing ceremony or just come out for his speech. We guessed the latter.

We told the Secretary's people of our plans to fill the DMZ with a complex series of zigzagging metal barriers, arranged to prevent all but an Olympic steeplechaser from reaching the stage. We would drape the four-foot-high barriers with fabric, and a few police officers would be hiding beneath the drapes like juvenile hide-and-go-seekers. We felt reasonably secure that the activists would not mount the stage.

But the barriers would separate Sullivan from the activists by only twenty or thirty feet, and we knew the "steeples" would be ringed with activists as soon as the Secretary rose to speak. The idea of placing a shield in front of the podium was rejected—Sullivan did not want to appear intimidated. We resolved that as the din in the hall became louder, we would simply turn up the sound system.

The question on everyone's mind, of course, was how to react if the situation deteriorated and violence appeared likely. Commander Tom Murphy of the SFPD was intent on avoiding mass arrests inside the hall—the police had been getting good reviews all week for their responsible handling of the demonstrations and did not want to jeopardize this at the eleventh hour. "We are not going to arrest people just for making noise," Murphy said. "We'll arrest them only if they try to climb over the barriers." We asked Bob Schmermund, one of Sullivan's press men, how important it was for Dr. Sullivan to address the conference.

"The Secretary really wants to give the speech," he said. "The speech lasts about twenty minutes, but can be divided up into parts and shortened if need be. This is what he'll do if he feels like he wants to leave. But his intent is to give the speech."

The discussion turned to timing. Although our original schedule called for Sullivan to be followed by Dr. Giovanni

Rossi, Chair of the 1991 conference in Florence, we increasingly felt that Rossi's welcoming words, like a gentle breeze following a tornado, would go unnoticed. We moved the Italian to earlier in the program, so that Sullivan's talk—and its reception—would, for all intents and purposes, end the conference. This meant that Sullivan's appearance at the podium was now scheduled for 12:15 P.M.; his handlers fretted about this timing in relation to the Gay and Lesbian Freedom Day Parade, still harboring the nightmarish vision of hundreds of thousands of angry gays storming the Moscone Center. Although the parade was scheduled to begin at 11:00 A.M., they knew that it traditionally ran late. "What time do you expect the thing to really begin?" nervously asked one of Sullivan's security men.

All eyes turned to Woodie Tennant, one of the "gay-sensitive" police in the SFPD contingent. A mischievous grin came over his face. "As soon as brunch is over," he said.

I was genuinely surprised when the closing ceremony party took the stage, and Secretary Sullivan, who had arrived earlier with an army of security men and reporters, strode to his seat. He had decided to sit through the entire ceremony.

Sullivan looked calm as he sat in his leather swivel chair surveying the audience. But the calm was studied; when I walked up to Volberding, sitting next to Sullivan on stage, to deliver a message, the Secretary saw something approach from the corner of his eye and literally jumped in his seat. I apologized, and slunk off stage. Sullivan regained his poise and settled back to listen.

The travel issue, so central in the opening ceremony, had been dormant during the bulk of the conference, finally overshadowed by scientific presentations. In fact, no conference-goers had been turned back at U.S. borders, and no gay visitors had challenged the Immigration Service. But, as Sullivan listened to speakers such as outgoing President of the International AIDS Society Lars Kallings and WHO Director-

General Hiroshi Nakajima, the travel issue made a rousing comeback.

"How can we expect the private person to behave in a rational and responsible way to prevent HIV infection or to reject prejudice when states set a bad example by instituting irrational laws and then, even worse, after realizing that the laws are unscientific and useless, through political bigotry do not change them?" asked Kallings.

"IAS resolves that further IAS-sponsored conferences will not be held in countries that restrict the entry of HIV-infected travelers. Therefore, IAS resolves to withdraw sponsorship from the Eighth International Conference on AIDS in Boston if U.S. immigration policy continues to restrict the travel of HIV-infected persons." Kallings's proclamations were met with loud cheers from the audience—cheers whose boisterousness and volume bespoke a far larger activist presence than earlier in the conference.

So focussed were the activists on Sullivan that only scattered chants of "Bring back Jonathan Mann" greeted Hiroshi Nakajima as he took the podium. But soon, the audience cheered as he too pounded away at the travel theme.

"I decided to come to San Francisco despite the travel restrictions because of the importance WHO attaches to these conferences, and to make clear WHO's position on freedom of international travel for HIV-infected persons," said the Director-General in halting English. "History has shown that the sudden appearance of any new disease can bring great misunderstanding and prejudice. . . . WHO looks forward to the day when future international conferences will not have to deal with discrimination in any form. To deal effectively and fully with this pandemic, we need solidarity and unity."

Finally, Giovanni Rossi, Chair of the Florence conference, welcomed the delegates to the Seventh International Conference on AIDS. He projected a slide of his historic and romantic city. "This is Florence," he said, "the most enjoyable, hospitable, and beautiful city in the world"—evoking some good-natured jeers from chauvinistic San Franciscans in the crowd—"always open to everyone who comes!"

Louis Sullivan listened dispassionately as the activists in the audience cheered louder and louder with each salvo launched at the government he represented. Dr. Anthony Fauci, the top AIDS official at the National Institutes of Health, spoke next. He was in a unique position to try to prevent the disaster he knew was coming, and so he tried.

Fauci had a longer, richer history with AIDS activism than anyone in the scientific community. As Director of the National Institute of Allergy and Infectious Diseases, the NIH agency charged with directing the AIDS research agenda, he had been vilified early and often by the activists.

At a 1987 speech in Boston, Larry Kramer described Fauci to a crowd of activists: "He's real cute. He's an Italian from Brooklyn, short, slim, compact; he wears aviator glasses and is a natty dresser, a very energetic and dynamic man. After a recent meeting a bunch of us from New York had with him, during which absolutely nothing was accomplished, he asked me what we thought of the meeting. I told him: 'Everyone thought you were real cute.' And he blushed to his roots. . . .

"You are smiling," Kramer upbraided the crowd, "and this is the man who has more effect on your future than anyone else, and he is not spending that forty-seven million dollars —*which was given to him specifically to test AIDS drugs*— and you are smiling!"

Another attack came after Fauci admitted to Congress that bureaucratic delays had set back the testing of aerosolized pentamidine, a drug eventually shown to prevent pneumocystis pneumonia in HIV-infected people.

"I have been screaming at the National Institutes of Health since I first visited your Animal House of Horrors in 1984," wrote Kramer in a 1988 open letter to Fauci. "ACT UP was formed over a year ago to get experimental drugs into the bodies of patients. For one year, ACT UP has tried every kind of protest known to man (short of putting bombs in your toilet or flames up your Institute) to get some movement in this area. One year later, ACT UP is still screaming for the same drugs they begged and implored you and your world to release. One year of screaming, protesting, crying, cajoling, lobbying, threatening, imprecating, marching, testifying, hoping, wishing, praying has brought nothing. You don't listen. No one listens. No one has ears. Or hearts. . . .

"All your 'doctors' have, continuously, told the world that All Is Being Done That Can Be Done. Now you admit that isn't so.

"WHY DID YOU KEEP QUIET FOR SO LONG?!

"I don't know (though it wouldn't surprise me) if you kept quiet intentionally. I don't know (though it wouldn't surprise me) if you were ordered to keep quiet by Higher Ups Somewhere and you are a good lieutenant, like Adolf Eichmann."

After years of these and other diatribes, by 1990 the landscape had changed. To the chagrin of more than a few scientists, Fauci had broken bread with the activists and profoundly altered his approach to AIDS drug testing. In an Afterword to his 1989 book *Reports from the holocaust*, Kramer sounded a rare conciliatory note.

"I would like to convey a special note of thanks to someone whom I criticized most severely in these pages, Dr. Anthony Fauci," wrote Kramer. "In crusading for the notion of 'parallel track'—a plan for making experimental drugs available while they are still in [FDA testing]—he has indeed become the 'hero' George Bush once named him. I now salute him, as must we all. It takes great courage for someone to alter so radically his position, admit he's wrong, and so energetically (and radically—Tony now sounds like a member of ACT UP) start out on a new path—a path that is also inherently critical of the work of his fellow bureaucrats."

Fauci was greeted warmly by the scientists and activists in the audience as he took the microphone. He had specifically told me that he wanted to speak about science and not politics, and did so for the first three-quarters of his talk. But the chance to send a message to the activists—and the scientists—before the coming eruption was irresistible.

"AIDS in the 1980s has revolutionized the relationship between the public and the scientists involved in AIDS research," Fauci said. "We are often confronted with the accusation by some that we are not doing enough and that we are moving too slowly. The scientific process which is the code of our professional existence is often seen as overly restrictive and even an impediment to solutions. Adherence to a set of scientific principles is often interpreted as insensitivity.

"The most vocal, provocative, and articulate groups are the AIDS activists. You heard from Peter Staley representing ACT UP New York in the opening ceremony [speaking] in an eloquent, passionate, angry, and poignant way of his personal fears and frustrations and the frustrations of his activist colleagues. They do have something important to say, and they can contribute constructively to our mission. . . .

"In the interactions between physician/scientists and activists, mistakes have been made by both sides. Activists are mistaken when they assume, or at least publicly state, that scientists do not care about them. Most scientists care deeply and are employing all of their energies and talents to accomplish the same goals as the activists. . . .

"It is particularly devastating and unfair when scientists of good faith and enormous talent are singled out and publicly named as scoundrels. I am not talking about myself, since it is part of my job, in one of the hats that I wear as a science administrator, to accept public criticism. I am referring to those individuals who devote themselves entirely to basic and clinical research. Besides, I have been vilified by the very best; I got my training with the godfather of vilification, Larry Kramer! . . .

"The challenge for scientists and science policymakers in the 1990s, as important as any specific project, is to display understanding, sensitivity, flexibility, and accessibility to the people who criticize us at the same time as we follow the paths down which our science leads us. As scientists, we are professionals fighting an intense war against a terrible disease. We are led by a quest for new knowledge and a desire to help mankind by solving problems critical to the public health. This is the way we serve. But we must never lose sight of the fact that the people whom we serve are the HIV-infected people throughout the world."

Even as Fauci spoke about cooperation and understanding, hundreds of activists streamed through the audience distributing a yellow flyer. NO MORE WORDS—WE WANT ACTION, it said boldly. Beneath, the text was chilling:

> Thus far during this conference, ACT UP has made many points *without disrupting the exchange of scientific information.* However, today's scheduled speech by Secretary of Health and Human Services, Dr. Louis B. Sullivan, is not a scientific presentation. After 10 years of Bush/Reagan rhetoric on AIDS, we will no longer tolerate words without action.
>
> You will not hear Louis Sullivan today.

Paul Volberding walked nervously to the microphone. "Our next speaker has been anticipated by all of us," he said. "In the spirit of the conference, and in the interest of the dialogue that we hope can continue from this conference, I welcome"—an audible gulp—"the Honorable Louis Sullivan, Secretary of Health and Human Services."

As soon as Volberding said the name "Sullivan," the Moscone Center was transformed into Times Square at midnight on New Year's Eve. A deafening roar of shouts, whistles, and air horn blasts consumed the hall as many in the audience of six thousand pressed their fingers to their ears. More than five hundred activists sprinted to the draped barricades, turned their backs on Sullivan, and raised banners. The largest one said simply: HE TALKS, WE DIE.

The Health Secretary sat in his seat for eight minutes, taking in the pandemonium. Then slowly, defiantly, he walked to the podium. Impossibly, the din grew louder.

"It is a great honor to spend a few moments with you," he began. The crowd began chanting, "Shame! Shame!"

"Let us not turn our frustrations into theater, searching for protagonists and antagonists. As scientists, advocates, and policymakers, we cannot become symbols driven by slogans, using the media as a proxy to provide high drama.

"The truth of the matter is that we need each other. And that will always be so. Until we can completely unravel the mysteries of this disease, we must find the ways and the means to work together." The chanting grew ever louder, the flyers were now paper airplanes launched at the podium. Within the hall, no one could decipher a word the Secretary was saying, and many were struck by the bizarre experience of watching his lips move without hearing his voice. Next to Sullivan, the signer for the hearing-impaired continued her efforts; ironically, her clients were the only ones in the hall destined to "hear" the speech.

Sullivan criticized the Chapman amendment, which would have allowed restaurants to exclude HIV-infected people from working as food handlers. AIDS advocates and scientists, citing the absence of evidence of HIV spread through food handling, had strongly attacked the amendment. "Any policy based on fears and misperceptions about HIV will only complicate and confuse disease control efforts without adding any protection to the public health," said Sullivan. But there was not a word about U.S. travel restrictions, a policy that failed to meet this very standard.

"Our frustrations must never drive us to close our ears or our hearts. Instead, AIDS must bring us together." Sirens began to wail through the hall, and our sound technicians turned up Sullivan's microphone. The result was increasing cacophony. Many of the clever ACT UPers weren't bothered, though: They had planned ahead and wore earplugs.

The activists began to toss more objects at the stoic Secretary, first wads of paper, then condoms, then bottles of cheap perfume. A few counterfeit conference identification badges were also tossed; artistically inclined activists had labored long into the night printing and laminating convincing forgeries, accounting for the surge in the activist presence. In the turbulent sea of protestors at Sullivan's feet, the noise grew louder, the anger more palpable. The Secretary was struck by one projectile, then another. "Why the hell don't they pull him before we have a riot?" I said under my breath. But Sullivan was hell-bent to finish.

"Let us stand together, united in common cause, because in the last analysis, that is what this conference is all about, and that must be our common declaration as the conference concludes. Thank you, and Godspeed in your work."

Louis Sullivan shook my hand as he left the stage—I saw only anger in his eyes—and sprinted to his waiting limousine. Reporters flocked to Sullivan's press secretary, Kay James, for reaction. The preplanned spin was ready. "It showed extraordinary courage by the Secretary to speak," she said. "It showed his commitment. His message is: 'I will not be silenced on this issue.' "

Meanwhile, the activists moved en masse out of the hall, the din gradually fading away like a police siren. The ACT UPers, media-savvy as always, were ready with their counterspin. "We are not going to stand for lip service anymore," said ACT UP's Josh Gamson. "We are demanding action, and we're not going to listen to any more empty rhetoric."

In the back of the hall, Jonathan Mann slowly shook his

head as the construction crews began to dismantle the stage in preparation for Moscone's next event. "The protestors missed a great opportunity to stand in silent protest and turn their backs," he said. "It was a sad demonstration."

"The image that will go out around the world is of a man speaking quietly, with dignity, in front of a wild crowd."

A few blocks away, the largest-ever Gay and Lesbian Freedom Day Parade had begun. The parade, as always, was joyous and informal. It began in traditional fashion with the ever-popular Dykes on Bikes, a pack of lesbians on motorcycles gunning their engines and baring their breasts to hundreds of thousands of cheering admirers—gay and straight alike. The procession passed bright rainbow-colored flags in window after window, symbolizing unity within the gay community. Though ACT UP had a presence, it was paltry compared to that of the flamboyant transvestites, the politicians, and the AIDS service organizations who have come to dominate the yearly event.

The loudest applause, observed Phil Hilts in the *New York Times*, was reserved for these AIDS service providers: ".·. . the volunteers who do laundry and run errands for the sick and the dying, the nurses and orderlies on the AIDS ward at San Francisco General Hospital, the hospice that rents a cable car each year to carry the weakest patients along the half-mile parade route."

14 BEYOND SAN FRANCISCO

The closing of the conference was a singularly abrupt experience, like the hours following an election. Suddenly, at 12:42 P.M. on Sunday, June 24, 1990, the big top came down and the circus moved to another town. A few days before the conference, our phones were lit like Christmas trees; someone trying to speak with me needed to successfully bypass five assistants. When we returned to our conference offices, however, I prayed for the receptionist to go to lunch so that I could answer the occasional phone call. Things were returning to normal; my Warholian fifteen minutes had come to an end.

A part of me ached at the conference's passing. It had all been so global and visible, so important and exhausting. And so seductive. This part of me watched with envy as several of our staff members left for Florence to begin work on the 1991 conference.

The envy was short-lived, since another part of me—one that had lain dormant for over a year—hungered for the return of life on a more human scale: caring for my patients, teaching a new and eager batch of students, becoming reacquainted with my family and friends. Over time I decompressed, and the tumult was replaced by a cache of indelible memories.

My fondest memories were of the team that worked together to plan the conference. Watching our people—one by one—pack their things and move on made the postpartum period especially sad. Dana Van Gorder, who had organized—through sheer force of personality—an international lobbying effort to change United States immigration policy, moved to the bohemian coastal town of Santa Cruz to manage a local political campaign. Paul Volberding succeeded Lars Kallings as IAS president, adding one more daunting responsibility to his extraordinary duties as clinician, researcher, and administrator. John Ziegler, for whom the conference caused a fundamental transformation from apolitical scientist to genuine AIDS advocate, left on a long-planned trip to direct a series of HIV drug trials in Uganda. Daily, another person who had invested their heart and soul in an effort that had often seemed futile entered my office to say good-bye. "Well, we did it," they would invariably say.

And indeed we had. Although we'd been dealt a stacked deck of cards, we had played it with skill and compassion, balancing the human, social and scientific needs of our impossibly diverse audience. While some reviewers focussed narrowly on the Sullivan episode (one sharp-witted scribe called it "the ultimate 'Read my lips' speech"), most took a broader perspective. "The events at the end of the closing were not able to touch the essence of the conference—which was the extraordinarily successful exchange of information," Jonathan Mann wrote us. "You have literally saved the future of the AIDS conferences, and thereby helped to rescue the solidarity we need from the people who, for whatever reason, commit actions which may tend to split us apart."

From the press also came kudos. "The thousands of voices in the halls and the streets around the Sixth International Conference on AIDS," wrote Lisa Levitt Ryckman of Associated Press, "resonated with passionate humanity, human compassion and intense dedication, love, anger, and grief. . . . The sounds of those voices linger in the memories of those who listened."

Unfortunately, the solidarity of the coalition continues to be threatened on a number of fronts. Within the activist movement, the issue of strategy is a major source of contention. ACT UP has been frankly surprised by its own success, and a bit unsure of how to handle it. Having gained access to the inner sanctum of power, what now?

Some argue, as I do, that collaboration with scientists and policymakers is necessary and proper. Within ACT UP, members of the Treatment and Data Committees such as New York's Mark Harrington and San Francisco's Jesse Dobson maintain that real change requires working with the system and breaking bread with the enemy. The parallel track concept, which blossomed from meetings between activists and federal scientists, is evidence of the utility of the collaborative approach. So too, I believe, was the success of the conference.

But others see things differently. Waiyde Palmer, representing a competing philosophy within ACT UP, said, "I have morals and ethics that run my life, no matter what my health status. I refuse to write off the needs of women and people of color, just so my needs can be met." This camp argues for a broader agenda: a full scale attack on racism, sexism, and homophobia at their roots, rather than a narrow focus on hastening scientific progress against AIDS.

As ACT UP's internal debate over political philosophy heats up, the need for consensus may render the group divided, paralyzed, and impotent. A case in point: ACT UP San Francisco split into two factions soon after the conference over this question of focus. Although other ACT UP chapters have not taken this radical step, the philosophical divide is ubiquitous.

Fueling the debate over strategy is the issue raised so acutely by Larry Kramer: the role of aggression. Even short of riots, many have noted an increased stridency to recent ACT UP actions, more "guerrilla" and less "theater." "There is a fine line between, on the one hand, street theater, civil disobedience, and the right to demonstrate, and on the other, mob behavior and brownshirting," wrote Tim Vollmer in the *San Francisco Sentinel*, a gay newspaper. "Many fear that the politics of anger is causing the community to abandon its commitment to the freedom of expression and the right to privacy, the two ideas used most often to support gay rights."

Most troubling is the specter of violence itself. To have dying people, bereft of hope, being exhorted by charismatic leaders to take up arms is a blueprint for disaster. One day someone may listen, and the damage to the cause will be irreparable. We can only pray that Larry Kramer refocuses his considerable rhetorical skills and passion in a more constructive direction.

But there are dangers in a kinder and gentler ACT UP as well. The fuel that drives the activists is unbridled anger. This has made them unpredictable, but also exceptionally effective, energizing the movement with an intensity not seen since the antiwar protests of the 1960s. When channeled constructively, the anger works—it stimulates a stagnant system in ways that genteel dialogue never could. Just as fanatical extremism will not further ACT UP's goals, neither will extreme mellowness.

In fact, as difficult as they often made my life, I came to value the activists as an essential element in the conference. Once given the stage, they and the people with AIDS who spoke were uniformly moving, perceptive, and provocative, adding an urgency and poignancy that would have otherwise been lacking. When I became frustrated by the street theater, I tried to remember something that ACT UP knows full well: Had we not feared disruption of our sessions, we would not have provided them a forum.

The forum permitted the birth of a coalition, one that held until the appearance of Louis Sullivan. The eruption was predictable. ACT UP's most valued currency is rage; the group could never allow itself to be seen as co-opted through the entire conference. Its members are understandably incensed over the timidity with which the government that Sullivan represents approaches AIDS, continuously protecting its flanks from conservative backlash. Perhaps the restraint shown at the meeting by ACT UP—not targeting working scientists, eschewing violence, waiting until the conference's waning moments to erupt—was the best we could hope for under the challenging circumstances.

The onus for nurturing the coalition is not on the activists alone. Scientists working in AIDS have an obligation to their patients and their research subjects. Part of this obligation is a moral one: We serve as our patients' agents, and must do all we can to protect their interests. And part of the obligation is practical: AIDS scientists owe much of their funding to the efforts undertaken on our behalf by AIDS advocates.

As we learned from planning the conference, scientists today must understand the politics of the epidemic, appreciating the anger and frustration driving the AIDS community. Patients demand that we explain what we do and why we do it, and they deserve answers. We need to convincingly argue that our primary motivation is not greed or self-advancement, but a genuine desire to help. The epidemic of mistrust can be stemmed, but it will take continued effort on our part to listen and be responsive to the communities we serve.

On the other hand, we must never sacrifice our scientific credibility for the sake of political expediency. At times, AIDS advocates may push us to do things we know not to be in the best interest of our patients. At these times, we must defend our position, articulating our stand without arrogance or paternalism, hoping that the community will understand, and never closing our ears and hearts to their concerns. We may take some heat from the advocacy community when we refuse to bow to the winds of protest, and this will be unpleasant. But credibility, once lost, is terribly hard to resurrect.

Our work with the Community Task Force is eloquent evidence that the product is worth the struggle. The Task Force, though born of political correctness and expediency, became a valued partner in every aspect of the conference. AIDS patients and their advocates demand such partnership; a "Task Force" is available to every scientist and physician working in the epidemic. Rather than feeling threatened, we should embrace this partnership, one that offers synergistic power far greater than the sum of its disparate parts.

Ironically, the success we had in forging a coalition was, I think, directly attributable to our two biggest headaches: the U.S. policy on HIV travel, and Larry Kramer. As committed as we were to tilling common ground between the scientists and activists, we would never have been able to do it without the travel issue. It rendered the scientists and activists bedfellows in their opposition to a mistaken policy and forced them to recognize their common interests, in a way that lofty calls to respect the sanctity of science could never have done. It also focussed the activists on a single issue—one that enjoyed broad support within the international scientific community—rather than a fragmented and contentious potpourri of empowerment struggles and parochial concerns.

Similarly, Larry Kramer's call for riots forced the activist community to examine the appropriateness of both their targets and their tactics. Had Kramer been mute, I fear the community would have remained splintered, a small minority opting to attack the scientists, perhaps even violently. When I saw the words "ACT UP has made many points without disrupting the exchange of scientific information" on ACT UP's closing ceremony flyer, I gave a silent thanks to Larry Kramer, brooding three thousand miles away, without whom such restraint would have been impossible.

Drug testing, access to care, research priorities, health-care worker issues—the epidemic provides a surfeit of opportunities for the coalition to mobilize and act. The alliance finally forged after a decade of this disease has demonstrated that scientists and activists can listen to one another and work together. The din during the closing ceremony could not drown out the harmonic swell of this collaboration.

POSTSCRIPT

E ven after the conference ended, the fight over the HIV travel issue continued. The organizers of the 1992 Boston conference and the members of the AIDS lobby carried the battle from San Francisco to the halls of Congress. The stakes were high. The Boston organizers and the International AIDS Society had committed themselves to moving the conference out of the U.S. if the policy wasn't fixed by the end of the 101st Congressional Session in October 1990. No action by Congress would mean that the San Francisco meeting would be the last held on American soil.

On October 25, 1990, at the literal eleventh hour, House and Senate negotiators approved an addition to a popular immigration bill moving briskly through Congress, one that both lifted the McCarthy-era ban on homosexual immigration and gave Health Secretary Sullivan the power to review and revise the list of "dangerous and contagious diseases." Just as in 1987, when Jesse Helms tacked the HIV-travel restrictions to a popular AZT funding bill, the marriage of the bills ensured prompt passage of the overall measure.

Had the travel restrictions remained intact and the 1992 conference moved out of the United States, one more vital coalition—that linking the American and international AIDS communities—would have been torn apart. Everyone in the AIDS world cheered the bill's passage, made possible by the unprecedented union between scientists and activists.

But the man who began the fight, Hans Paul Verhoef, could not join in the celebration. On July 23, 1990, he died at his home in Delft, Holland. Hans Paul Verhoef was thirty-three years old.

As always in AIDS, milestones and tombstones are tragic partners.

APPENDIX 1:
CAST OF CHARACTERS

Art Agnos, Mayor of San Francisco.

Dr. James Allen, Director of the National AIDS Program Office of the U.S. Public Health Service.

Duke Austin, spokesman for the U.S. Immigration and Naturalization Service.

Jack Ballentine, conference security consultant.

Paul Boneberg, member of the conference's Community Task Force, and Director of San Francisco's Mobilization Against AIDS.

Jim Bunn, conference communications director.

Larry Bush, assistant for gay community affairs to San Francisco Mayor Art Agnos.

Al Casciato, conference security consultant.

Pat Christen, member of the conference's Community Task Force, and Executive Director of the San Francisco AIDS Foundation.

Dr. Ellen Cooper, AIDS drug regulator at the U.S. Food and Drug Administration.

Martin Delaney, conference speaker, and Director of San Francisco's Project Inform.

David Demarest, Director of Communications in the Bush White House.

Dr. Anthony Fauci, Director of the National Institute of Allergy and Infectious Diseases at the U.S. National Institutes of Health.

Alan Fein, Executive Director of the Eighth International Conference on AIDS, Boston, Massachusetts.

Dr. Margaret Fischl, Director of AIDS Research at the University of Miami.

Jim Foster, veteran gay activist and member of the San Francisco Health Commission.

Debra Fraser-Howze, conference speaker, and Director of New York's Black Leadership Coalition on AIDS.

Dr. George Galasso, Chair of the Third International Conference on AIDS, Washington, D.C.

Dr. Robert Gallo, retrovirologist at the U.S. National Cancer Institute.

Alixe Glen, Deputy Press Secretary in the Bush White House.

Shirley Gross, Cochair of the conference's Community Task Force, and Director of San Francisco's Bayview–Hunter's Point Foundation, a minority advocacy group.

Mark Harrington, conference speaker, and member of ACT UP New York's Treatment and Data Committee.

Dennis Hartzell, director of fundraising for the conference.

Ivan Head, Chair of the Fifth International Conference on AIDS, Montreal, Canada.

U.S. Senator Jesse Helms, conservative Senator who authored the 1987 law restricting the entry of HIV-infected people to the United States.

Philip Hilts, AIDS and health care reporter for the *New York Times*.

Dr. Dan Hoth, Director of the Division of AIDS at the National Institute of Allergy and Infectious Diseases at the U.S. National Institutes of Health.

Michael Iskowitz, Assistant to Senator Edward Kennedy on the U.S. Senate Committee on Labor and Human Relations.

Dr. Stephen Joseph, former New York City Health Commissioner.

Dr. Lars Olof Kallings, President of the International AIDS Society.

Kathleen Kay, Jonathan Mann's assistant at the Global Programme on AIDS of the World Health Organization.

Eunice Kiereini, keynote speaker in the conference's opening ceremony, and Chair of Family Health, Foundation of Kenya.

Larry Kramer, New York novelist and playwright, founder of ACT UP, and cofounder of the Gay Men's Health Crisis.

Pierre Ludington, member of the conference's Community Task Force, and Executive Director of the American Association of Physicians for Human Rights.

Dr. Jonathan Mann, former Director of the Global Programme on AIDS, World Health Organization.

Dr. James Mason, U.S. Assistant Secretary of Health.

Jean McGuire, Executive Director of the AIDS Action Council, a Washington, D.C., AIDS lobbying group.

Dr. Leon McKusick, Cochair of the conference's Community Task Force, and a psychologist in San Francisco's gay community.

Dr. Luc Montagnier, retrovirologist at Paris's Pasteur Institute, head of the team that first isolated the AIDS virus.

Dr. Steve Morin, member of the conference's Community Task Force, and Assistant to U.S. Representative Nancy Pelosi.

Dr. Hiroshi Nakajima, Director-General of the World Health Organization.

Dr. June Osborn, Chair of the U.S. National Commission on AIDS.

Sallie Perryman, speaker in the conference's opening ceremony, and an AIDS advocate employed by the AIDS Institute for New York State.

Dr. Arnold Relman, conference speaker, and Editor of the *New England Journal of Medicine.*

Dr. Giovanni Rossi, Chair of the Seventh International Conference on AIDS, Florence, Italy.

Vito Russo, originally chosen to speak in the conference's opening ceremony, a New York writer and member of ACT UP.

Randy Shilts, AIDS political journalist, author of *And the Band Played On.*

Michael Shriver, member of the conference's Community Task Force, and a member of ACT UP and San Francisco's 18th Street Services.

Dr. Mervyn Silverman, President of the American Foundation for AIDS Research (AmFAR), and former San Francisco Health Director.

Peter Staley, speaker in the conference's opening ceremony, and a member of ACT UP New York.

Dr. Louis Sullivan, U.S. Secretary of Health and Human Services.

U.S. Attorney General Richard Thornburgh, Director of the Justice Department, which oversees the Immigration and Naturalization Service.

Dana Van Gorder, Press and Community Relations Director of the Sixth International Conference on AIDS.

Hans Paul Verhoef, AIDS educator who first challenged the U.S. Immigration Service's restrictions on travel by HIV-infected people.

Dr. Paul Volberding, Cochair of the Sixth International Conference on AIDS.

Dr. Robert Wachter, Program Director of the Sixth International Conference on AIDS.

U.S. Representative Henry Waxman, Chair of the House Subcommittee on Health and the Environment.

Dr. John Ziegler, Chair of the Sixth International Conference on AIDS.

APPENDIX 2:
HISTORY OF THE
INTERNATIONAL
CONFERENCES ON AIDS

1985	First International Conference on AIDS	Atlanta, Georgia, U.S.A.
1986	Second International Conference on AIDS	Paris, France
1987	Third International Conference on AIDS	Washington D.C., U.S.A.
1988	Fourth International Conference on AIDS	Stockholm, Sweden
1989	Fifth International Conference on AIDS	Montreal, Canada
1990	Sixth International Conference on AIDS	San Francisco, California, U.S.A.
1991	Seventh International Conference on AIDS	Florence, Italy*
1992	Eighth International Conference on AIDS	Boston, Massachusetts, U.S.A.*
1993	Ninth International Conference on AIDS	Berlin, Germany*

*planned

APPENDIX 3:
ONE DAY IN THE LIFE OF THE SIXTH INTERNATIONAL CONFERENCE ON AIDS

Friday, June 22, 1990

MORNING PLENARY SESSIONS (8:00 – 10:30 A.M.)

STATE OF THE ART SESSION ("SCIENTIFIC"): EPIDEMIOLOGY AND BASIC RESEARCH

The Prevention of HIV Infection in Injecting Drug Users: Recent Advances and Remaining Obstacles
Gerry V. Stimson
Director, The Centre for Research on Drugs and Health Behaviour, United Kingdom

SCIENCE TO POLICY SESSION ("ISSUES"): CLINICAL TRIALS AND DRUG DEVELOPMENT

Approaches to Drug Development
George Gill
Director, Drug and Regulatory Affairs
Bristol Myers-Squibb, U.S.A.

Evolution of Clinical Trials Design
Peter Armitage
Oxford University, United Kingdom

Changing Demographics of
HIV Infection in Latin
America
Jaime Sepulveda
Director General of
Epidemiology, Mexico

Epidemiology and Primary
Prevention of HIV
Infection in Adolescents
Mindy Fullilove
HIV Center for Clinical and
Behavioral Studies
New York State Psychiatric
Institute/Columbia
University, U.S.A.

Immune Response to HIV
Andrew McMichael
John Radcliffe Hospital,
Oxford University, United
Kingdom

Vaccine Approaches Against
HIV
Jay Berzofsky
National Cancer Institute,
U.S.A.

Animal Models of
Lentivirus Infection
Murray Gardner
Department of Pathology
University of California,
Davis, U.S.A.

Progress in AIDS Clinical
Trials
Dan Hoth
Director, Division of AIDS
National Institute of Allergy
and Infectious Diseases,
U.S.A.

Alternatives to Traditional
Trials: Community
Contribution
Martin Delaney
Executive Director, Project
Inform, U.S.A.

AIDS Clinical Trials: The
Perspective of
Communities of Color
Debra Fraser-Howze
Executive Director and
CEO
Black Leadership
Commission on AIDS,
U.S.A.

Clinical Trials in the
Developing World
Elly Katabira
Mulago Hospital, Uganda

Reporting of Clinical Trials
Arnold Relman
Editor, New England
Journal of Medicine

MID-DAY POSTER SECTIONS (10:30 A.M. – 1 P.M.)

More than 700 posters (each a study depicted in graphic and text form on an eight-foot-wide by four-foot-high corkboard) dealing with:

Basic Science (Track A): HIV Replication, HIV Receptors and Tropism, Viral Pathogenesis, HIV Isolation and Detection, Evolutionary Relationship of the Immune-Deficiency Viruses;

Clinical Science and Trials (Track B): Neurology of AIDS, Clinical Heterogeneity, Pediatric and Obstetric AIDS, Nursing Research, Hematology/Immunology/Allergy, Miscellaneous Organ Systems;

Epidemiology and Prevention (Track C): HIV Seroprevalence in North America, Latin America, Africa, Asia, Europe, and Oceania; HIV-2 Seroprevalence; Modelling and Research Methods; Determinants of Risk Behaviors in Homosexual and Bisexual Men, Heterosexuals, and Drug Users; Projections and Estimates of HIV and AIDS;

Social Science and Policy (Track D): Community Organization and Advocacy, Cost and Financing, Resource Allocation, Cost Effectiveness of Early Drug Treatment, Media and the Dissemination of Information, National and International Programs and Policies.

AFTERNOON ORAL SESSIONS (1:00 – 3:00 P.M. and 3:30 – 5:30 P.M)

Basic Science (Track A): Advances in HIV Vaccine Development, Related Retroviruses, Anti-Viral Drug Development, Cellular Immunity in HIV Infection;

Clinical Science and Trials (Track B): Anti-Retroviral Therapy in Children and Pregnant Women, Early Diagnosis and Treatment of Neurologic Disease, The Impact of Therapy on the Course of HIV Infection, Cytomegalovirus and Other Viral Opportunistic Infections;

Epidemiology and Prevention (Track C): Reducing Occupational Risks among Health Care Workers, Epidemiology of HIV and AIDS in the Developed World, Epidemiology of HIV and AIDS in the Developing World, Issues in Parenterally Transmitted HIV Infection;

Social Science and Policy (Track D): AIDS and the Media; National and International Programs and Policies; Community Organization and Activism; Cost, Financing, and Resource Allocation.

CONFERENCE EXHIBITS

Each day of the conference, more than 250 exhibitors displayed their wares. About half were commercial concerns, including major manufacturers of drugs, diagnostic tools, and condoms. A few were large government organizations, such as the Centers for Disease Control and the National Institutes of Health. Finally, about 120 were community-based organizations—ranging from large advocacy groups like the San Francisco AIDS Foundation and the American Foundation for AIDS Research to smaller organizations like Birmingham (Alabama) AIDS Outreach, the Haitian Coalition on AIDS, and Swedish Physicians Against AIDS.

COMMUNITY OUTREACH SESSIONS

These sessions were developed by the Community Task Force, and cosponsored by the conference, a number of local community groups, and the Levi Strauss Company. They were held in the evening at an off-conference site and were open free of charge to the community. Friday's session dealt with "Treatment, Research, and Clinical Trials," and featured Dr. Anthony Fauci of the NIH, Dr. Ellen Cooper of the FDA,

Martin Delaney of Project Inform, Mark Harrington of ACT UP New York, and a number of community representatives.

DEMONSTRATIONS

Friday's major demonstration dealt with women and AIDS, as 150 members of ACT UP's women's contingent staged a "die-in" in the middle of San Francisco's Market Street.

INDEX